'In *Glow*, beauty writer Vasudha Rai, who has previously worked as a beauty editor for magazines like *Harper's Bazaar India* and *Cosmopolitan India*, ignores trending buzzwords and attempts to simplify what should ideally be a straightforward return to natural beauty remedies. The book offers a concise summary of effective ingredients that live up to their promise of stress-reducing, gut-cleansing and skin-clearing benefits'—*Mint Lounge*

'As a certified yogi with over 15 years in the beauty business, Vasudha Rai helps clear the air in her debut book, *Glow*. She goes back to the basics of turmeric and ghee, and turns to Ayurveda to document Indian foods that can give you the best skin and hair of your life. Plus, there's a scientific and Ayurvedic explanation for each beauty food, along with a recipe on the best way to use it, so there's no questioning whether it really works'—*Vogue*

'Vasudha Rai's excellent book *Glow* is for people who have a million tabs open in their brain, but also want to be vaguely healthy. Yes it's a beauty book that celebrates what beauty should be—a holistic lifestyle that makes you feel good about yourself. It's also easy and accessible with ingredients and recipes that even kitchen-haters like me can attempt. My copy is comfortingly dog eared. It was the first thing I would pick up to read in the morning before the day attacked. And it was the best kind of start you could ask for. Positive, happy, doable, and most importantly, knowledgeable. The exhaustive research is so satisfying because of the way she's broken it down, making sure no matter what your concern, skin type or curiosity, you'll find a page, or 100, worth mulling over. Vasudha teaches you to take care of yourself, of how you look, with Indian herbs, leaves, shoots, grains and flowers, supported by nutritionists, doctors, Ayurvedic experts and beauty industry gurus. Make sure you buy two copies. Keep one for yourself and gift a "Glow" to a friend'—Rituparna Som, editor-in-chief, *VICE* India

'I loved reading the book. I believe so much in the same philosophy. I've been through my share of challenges health-wise and in life in general—like all of us—and every single time it's been old-fashioned Indian food and Ayurveda that have saved me. I love the way the book is structured and the information is so easy, but also completely new'—Chinmayee Manjunath, editor, book sherpa, content coach

'Most books which deal with holistic beauty, tend to slide into extreme territory, promoting unreasonable lifestyle choices, expensive superfoods, or unscientific theories about health. Beauty guru Vasudha Rai's offering *Glow*, wins one over first and foremost because it does none of those things. Balanced and well-researched, it presents readers with accessible ways to enhance the beauty within by making healthy choices . . . Very easy to read and uncomplicated, this book contains no flowery adjectives, complex language, or verbose sentences. Being so heavy on information, it is actually best in this format, letting the content do the work instead of the form. For a first-time author and long-time beauty editor for some of India's largest fashion magazines, this book is a huge win. For consumers of beauty and health content, this book is a treasure'—iDiva

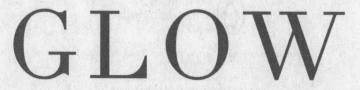

GLOW

*Indian Foods, Recipes and Rituals
for Beauty, Inside and Out*

VASUDHA RAI

Foreword by Masaba Gupta

EBURY
PRESS

An imprint of Penguin Random House

EBURY PRESS

USA | Canada | UK | Ireland | Australia
New Zealand | India | South Africa | China

Ebury Press is part of the Penguin Random House group of companies
whose addresses can be found at global.penguinrandomhouse.com

Published by Penguin Random House India Pvt. Ltd
7th Floor, Infinity Tower C, DLF Cyber City,
Gurgaon 122 002, Haryana, India

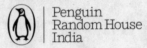

First published in Ebury Press by Penguin Random House India 2018

Copyright © Vasudha Rai 2018
Foreword copyright © Masaba Gupta 2018

Illustrations by Jit Chowdhury

All rights reserved

10 9 8 7 6 5

While every effort has been made to verify the authenticity of the information
contained in this book, it is not intended as a substitute for consultation with a
psychologist, nutritionist or dermatologist. The publisher and the author are
in no way liable for the use of the information contained in this book.

ISBN 9780143441595

Typeset in Adobe Garamond Pro by Manipal Digital Systems, Manipal
Printed at Replika Press Pvt. Ltd, India

This book is sold subject to the condition that it shall not, by way of trade
or otherwise, be lent, resold, hired out, or otherwise circulated without the
publisher's prior consent in any form of binding or cover other than that in
which it is published and without a similar condition including this condition
being imposed on the subsequent purchaser.

www.penguin.co.in

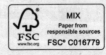

For Krishna Reya

दीपो भक्षयते ध्वान्तं कज्जलं च प्रसूयते ।
यदन्नं भक्षयेन्नित्यं जायते तादृशी प्रजा ॥

Dipo bhakshayate dhvantam kajjalam cha prasuyate
Yadannam bhakshayennityam jayate tadrishi praja

The lamp eats darkness and produces black soot. So
the quality of the food one eats daily determines what
one will produce. Meaning: You are what you eat.

—Chanakya, *Chanakya Shatakam*

CONTENTS

PART II: CLARITY

PART III: RADIANCE

PART IV: PEACE

FOREWORD

The interesting thing about beauty is that your ideas about it change as you grow older. When you're young, you want to look like your favourite actor, your mother or even an air hostess. That's because you don't have an opinion about how you look. The hardest years for beauty are adolescence. You don't know what's going to be a strength—all you see are flaws.

I feel so much more confident now, in my thirties. Just a few weeks ago I was in our holiday home in the hills and had a lot of time on my hands. After a shower I examined my body, which I usually don't do. I turned around and saw that I had scars all the way from my upper back to my hips. A thought crossed my mind about visiting a dermatologist, who would perhaps give me ten creams to apply. But then I thought: what's the point? That was the moment I realized I'm okay with this. I know that I have to take care of my body but I can't be worried about it each morning. It also comes from the fact that I'm in a marriage and I'm secure. It would perhaps make a difference when you're just about to date a man.

Beauty today has become a big burden instead of being something that should make you feel elevated. It has become a baggage because we have so many brands, products and expectations. And along with that, there are people's opinions—some that will teach you kindness and others that will tear you apart. And you pick up on each of these signals. No matter how much I write and how much I share, everyone has a different journey with beauty. You keep redefining your idea of it till the very end.

What my mom said ten years ago makes sense today. When we are young no one teaches us what true beauty really is—that behaviour and physicality are irrevocably intertwined. If you behave badly you look ugly no matter how perfect your features may be. Some people just look bitter and don't have a sparkle in their eyes. Their energy isn't half as beautiful as their physical appearance. I know people who are overweight who have faces full of scars, but they look beautiful to me because of the way they speak or behave.

When you're younger you judge people on their physical attributes but beauty is so much more than that. Physical beauty is superficial and it will always fade. You may want the person you marry to have a list of outward characteristics— the ideal height, body and skin—but once you exhaust that, what's next? You can't live with a shell of beauty that's empty inside. Sadly, we don't talk about this enough.

I saw that in myself. When I was thirteen or fourteen I had acne and braces. I also didn't like that I had curves. I felt that I looked horrible and because of that I was upset with everything. Today my basic structure is the same but I'm just happier because I have accepted a lot of who I am. When I meet girls I tell them that if they can come to terms with at least one flaw, they'll be much happier. But acceptance goes hand in hand with change. I became much calmer when my skin started clearing up. The funny thing is that as you grow older, you realize that there is a cure for everything, and that really helps you. You become calmer by finding solutions. I genuinely feel that I can talk so openly about it because I have found a solution. I wouldn't talk about it if I had a face full of acne.

The solution also comprises the right diet, sleep and exercise. Still I'm somebody who never denies myself anything. People who constantly worry about healthy food are more bitter. I've become very disciplined about my workout. My rule is 80–20—through the week I try and eat very well. But I eat whatever I want during the weekends, even if it's French fries for breakfast. When you work out, eat (mostly) right and sleep well, your face transforms. Especially when you exercise because the minute you sweat, everything just changes—it's an instant mood-booster.

For these reasons I feel a book like *Glow* is so relevant, because Vasudha stresses on the holistic idea of beauty that goes beyond physicality. And the great part is that she's talking about Indian ingredients. As Indians we still have a colonial hangover. But our home-grown foods are bursting with benefits. Even simple things like turmeric, clove and ginger have medicinal properties. This book has come out at the right time, because there's a big beauty revolution where all the conventional brands are facing stiff competition from traditional products. I, for example, use a face cleansing paste with moong dal in it.

Vasudha herself has obviously come a long way. I love to watch her videos because they're very simple yet detailed. She is also someone who practises what she preaches. She believes in wellness and I've seen that in the food she eats and the glow on her skin. She's certainly a flag-holder for what she writes about. She simplifies the idea of wellness but more than anything else she is India-proud, and that I feel is truly incredible.

Mumbai   Masaba Gupta
April 2018

INTRODUCTION

In the early 2000s, when the world stopped eating carbs, I started writing about beauty. In those days health and beauty were separate. You could even say that healthy people didn't care much about looking good. It was different from today, when we see beauty not as an indulgence but as an act of self-care—or at least we should.

In those days, most dermatologists in the country used to say that what we ate had no connection with how we looked. At that time there was no research to prove that skin and food were connected, so doctors relied only on creams and antibiotics to clear the complexion. And it wasn't any different for me. My primary focus was cosmetics. I used a serum to eliminate frizz, silicon-laden primers to make pores 'appear' smaller and benzoyl peroxide to shrink breakouts. I drank water sporadically; during the week or so that I made an effort to drink more H_2O, my skin and hair looked much better. But soon I was back to my old habits—less water, more sugar and cheese. Eventually it showed up in 2006 as grade-IV endometriosis.

Nobody knows why endometriosis really happens, and there's no real cure for it. After fighting it for more than a decade, with myriad combinations of allopathic medicines, I'm sure of one thing: stress and a poor diet are its main triggers. While medicine helped control the disease, it didn't completely reduce the symptoms, especially the pain. In the years after I was diagnosed, my concept of beauty changed. Rather than something purely cosmetic, I began to see it as holistic. Then, I discovered yoga.

I have been practising yoga for more than seven years now and I also teach. I don't think of it as a practice of asanas any more. Yoga is what I do when I am off my mat. Because it has built my awareness, I'm cognizant of everything I consume—be it the food I eat or the thoughts that run through my mind. I always ask myself two things: Is this useful, and is this worth it? I find that more than 90 per cent of what we think and what we want to eat is neither useful nor worth it. What goes on inside shows up on the outside. Good skin is just a symptom of great health.

Over the last fifteen years or so, I've tried and tested, tracked and followed every beauty, health and wellness trend. But nothing really was a revelation. Eating superfoods did not change my life, and fad diets made me petulant. With these experiences, I realized that the intuitive capabilities of the human mind are far greater than any wellness trend. Therefore, what really works is listening to your own body and respecting its signals. When you eat, observe not only how the food tastes on your tongue but also how it settles afterwards. Instead of following trends, decode your own internal language. When you remove the cobwebs from your mind, you can build your own rituals.

Today, we're fortunate to live in an age where wellness is the new currency of cool. But as it becomes the ultimate luxury, we've forgotten its first rule—simplicity.

While this new infatuation with self-care is well intended, it hasn't made health more accessible. Eating and living well has become an expensive proposition. Overpriced supplements, protein powders, green juices and nut butters are the new necessities. Everywhere you look, there are gluten-free pastas, packaged muesli, energy balls and kombucha—all with the promise to fill you to the brim with health. But gluten-free pasta is made with refined flour, and most packaged muesli is highly processed. Kombucha, in fact, is already facing a backlash in health circles because of its high sugar content. And, in truth, there's no better energy ball than a home-made laddu.

Before we dive into the world of beauty-bestowing ingredients, we must stop looking at foods as mere trends. Health is not a trend but a necessity. While skincare and make-up are accepted tools they should come last not first in the quest for beauty. The problem is that we leapfrog to embellishments and forget the basics. We eschew easily available food for novelty ingredients. I too went to great lengths to source the latest superfoods, paying enormous amounts in customs duties. It would have been impossible for me not to, especially because I test these things before writing about them.

The 'superfood' tag makes us undervalue everyday meals and pay extra for a health boost. But imagine the naivety of investing in imported elixirs when we live in the land of Ayurveda. India's rich heritage, traditions and mysticism are undisputed but our ultimate treasures are our precious foods, rituals and recipes. We have given the world yoga, fasting, turmeric, sandalwood, *ashwagandha* and ghee. What's exotic for them lies at our doorstep. In the next few years all health trends will come from our glorious country, be it *triphala*, millets or *chyawanprash*. It's now time to reclaim our knowledge and get reacquainted with our inheritance.

After many years of tinkering with new-age nutrition I have come to realize that what changes us is simple everyday food. We often skip the unglamorous bits for the 'Instagrammable' ones. But supplements, beauty powders and medicinal mushrooms only work when they're layered over wholesome meals. I love Indian food, cooked at home in local oils, using time-tested methods, with seasonal produce. After reading, writing and researching on food, I've learnt that our recipes aren't based on flavour alone. There's deep wisdom behind what's on the plate. Traditional Indian meals marry medicinal herbs with intense flavour. When I live in India I like to eat local, cooking with unrefined flours, oils and sugars.

We use these everyday ingredients for beauty rituals too. Our long-established oils and *ubtans*, made with lentils, grains, milk and honey, aren't just beautifying but sustainable too. A home-made bath powder does not pollute waterbodies nor is it expensive. I love good skincare products and luxurious make-up, and I also have a dermatologist on call. But I equally love traditional concoctions of hair oils, cleansers and masks. It's all about balance—moving forward, while being connected to our roots.

This book contains just a fraction of what to eat and apply. By no means are these foods superior to other fruits, vegetables or herbs. I have carefully chosen ingredients that I have loved. However, they are not the only ones to use because the more variety we eat, the more nutrients we get. Every food has its own unique combination of vitamins, minerals, antioxidants and fatty acids. When we eat fruits of different colours, rotate oils, mix nuts and temper with a multitude of spices, we reap maximum benefits. So, it would be unfair to limit ourselves to just this list.

I've also divided this book into what I consider to be the four pillars of beauty—vitality, clarity, radiance and peace. Beauty that exists in a vacuum for show value alone is pointless and ephemeral. While looking good is a big part of being beautiful, if it's the only dimension, it will lack depth and purpose. Instead, if we look at attractiveness from the lens of behaviour, health, energy and appearance, it will make everything more accessible, impactful and enduring.

Vitality is the first pillar because energy and strength— both inner and outer—lay the foundation for beauty. If our immunity is weak and we're always tired, how will we ever look good? The concept of delicate beauty is relevant only in fairy tales. Real beauties are spirited, determined and empowered. When we're physically and emotionally strong we make better decisions because we're energized with health. In this first part I present a collection of oils, grains, raw sugars and herbs that bestow you with vital energy.

We often hear that beauty is skin deep. I too believe that clear skin is its fundamental tenet. From a physical perspective, clarity is the first sign of inner health. When I was growing up I struggled with acne, and during those days the only wish I had was clear skin. After trying an assortment of treatments, I found that ultimately it's about what we eat. The second part, called clarity, holds a treasury of potent herbs and everyday vegetables that detoxify the body and purify your complexion.

After we gain spotless skin, we all aspire for radiance. In the third part I explore the real foundation for luminous skin—antioxidants that work like magnets to pull out toxins from our bodies. They work by neutralizing free radicals and removing toxic molecules that come from the environment and are produced internally because of stress. In this part I list the most salubrious Indian berries, healing greens, fragrant flowers and spices that light you up from within.

But the holy grail of beauty is peace within. To me it's the ultimate essential that augments all aspects of our looks and personality—because it's about not only how we look but also how we feel. Bliss has its own special aura. Forget about being attractive for other people. When you're calm, you look good to yourself. If you work on peace as a priority, it will illuminate you from within.

Even Maslow's Hierarchy of Human Needs has a five-tier system of requirements according to importance.[1] Once a certain need is fulfilled only then can we move to the next level. The foundation of this pyramid is built on food, water and safety. Once this is achieved, we look for friendship, love and self-esteem. And it's only when we're satisfied with these aspects that we can move to the last realm of self-actualization. If we work on ourselves in a similar fashion, moving from vitality, clarity and radiance towards peace, it holds the potential to change our lives. This is the ultimate path to everlasting beauty. This is how we *Glow*.

PART I

VITALITY

We operate out of two emotions—fear and love. Both sentiments make us truly human. However, they're the opposite of each other. When we work out of fear, the result is usually weak and lacklustre. But when we do something from a place of love, the results are inspirational. It's no different with food.

In today's world there's so much misplaced knowledge that we eat out of fear. Will this make me fat? Am I allergic to this? Should I feel guilty after an indulgence? With each bite we become more afraid, and consequently, our bodies shut down, refusing to accept nourishment. Even when we treat ourselves, we become overwhelmed with guilt, which prevents us from truly enjoying the moment. You see, it's not just what you eat that is important but also how you eat it. The more you relish your food, the more it will energize you.

Over the last few decades many trends have come and gone. First, fat was the enemy and now it's our best friend. Meat was also glorified for a brief moment, while carbs were pilloried for causing weight gain. After writing on health and beauty for many years, the only thing I've learnt is that today's remedy could be tomorrow's poison. Foods that nourish you greatly could be stigmatized because of new research. And ingredients that were considered poisonous may be celebrated again.

The problem begins when we focus just on the outward manifestation of beauty. When washboard abs become more important than an energized body, we fail in the quest for health. The perpetual obsession with superfoods takes away the pleasure of eating. It separates us from the time-tested knowledge of our ancestors. While traditions have always been relevant, you'll find that they are more applicable today than ever before. In fact, at a time when we're bombarded with a new trend every day, ancient, time-tested wisdom is worth our trust.

Vitality is the feeling of freshness, energy and strength. It helps us look forward to the day and handle each task with ease, including the chore of self-care. We need to be strong and energized first, before even thinking about the other aspects of beauty such as clarity and radiance. In this part we'll focus on the basics that make us robust—oils, grains, unrefined sugars and herbs—ingredients from our kitchens that must be included in our everyday diet.

I've included carbs and sugars in this selection because I don't believe in completely eliminating any food group. While I limit my consumption of wheat, milk and sugar because they cause inflammation, I haven't removed them entirely from my diet. It's essential to enjoy everything in moderation. Unless you're intolerant or allergic to any ingredient, there's really no reason to completely cut it out.

The need of the hour is to stop treating meals as a battlefield. We must eat with the aim of boosting health and longevity, instead of trying to create only the outward shell of a perfect body. After all, there can be outward beauty only when there's inner health.

1

GHEE

According to Vagbhata's *Ashtanga Samgraha*, one must look at his or her reflection in ghee before beginning the day. In earlier times, when there were no mirrors, it was advised that you should not look at your reflection in a dirty river or well. Ghee was considered to be the most sacred, purest ingredient, and therefore ideal to mirror your face.

My yoga guru, Seema Sondhi, eats a couple of teaspoons of ghee on an empty stomach each morning because she believes that this wonderful fat nourishes not just the bones, joints and skin, but also the *nadi*s in the body. Nadis refer both to the nerves as well as the energy channels or meridians (as the Chinese call them). We have about 72,000 nadis or energy channels, and about 95–100 billion neurons or nerve cells. Ghee, therefore, has both physical and spiritual significance because it nourishes both aspects.

We use ghee to purify the environment in pujas, weddings and havans. For us, in India, its benefits go beyond just bodybuilding. It is believed that just sprinkling ghee on food purifies the soul. In Haryana (from where I come) eating ghee is a no-brainer. Some of my vivid childhood memories are of enjoying rotis slathered with this divine fat and my brother drinking the ghee and then eating his roti. I cannot imagine a single meal without it because it just elevates the flavour and effect of food. My grandfather used to say that the only thing he carried from his village in Haryana to his college in Delhi was desi ghee. He died at the age of ninety-six, sharp as a tack, with all his hair and teeth intact.

Science

Ghee's strength-enhancing capabilities make it popular among athletes and yogis alike. It's no surprise then that when Haryana sportspeople won thirty-two medals for India at the Commonwealth Games in 2010, along with cash prizes, they were also gifted between 51–101 kg of ghee by the state's chief minister. Ghee nourishes and makes the connective tissue more elastic, boosts digestion and increases strength. It also lubricates the joints, so if you don't want joint problems as you grow older, make sure you include it in your diet.

One of its many wonderful properties is that it helps mobilize fat deposits. This means that it breaks down fatty pockets and evenly distributes weight, so you look more proportional. But don't think of it as an excuse to be lazy. Ghee is a fat, and without exercise it will increase weight. However, if you're active, it will help reduce weight or at the very least distribute it evenly.

We now know that the gut is the epicentre of good health. From digestion to weight, skin quality and even mood—it controls everything. Here, too, ghee has immense benefits. It is the highest source of butyric acid, a saturated short-chain fatty acid found in animal fat, wholegrains and vegetable oil. It's also produced by us internally, and is important because it ensures the health of our digestive system by being food for the cells in the colon.

Despite being a saturated fat, ghee is immensely healthy because it increases high-density lipoprotein (HDL, which pulls fat from the bloodstream) and reduces low-density lipoprotein (LDL, that sticks to the arteries). In addition, it's made of short-chain fatty acids that are easier to digest as compared to long-chain fatty acids found in butter. Ghee is also made up of 25–35 per cent monounsaturated fatty acids (MUFA), a healthy fat found in olive oil, avocados and nuts. Not only do MUFAs enhance cardiovascular health, they also benefit insulin and blood sugar levels. But wait, there's more. Ghee also contains a whopping amount of vitamins A, E and K, which are essential for beautiful skin and hair. The best part about this fat is that it doesn't contain either lactose or casein, which is why it can be consumed by those who are lactose-intolerant.

Ghee is also an internal cleanser. Detoxification mainly happens through the liver, which produces bile required by exotic oils (such as olive) to digest. But ghee and coconut oil don't require bile. Therefore, these fats, unlike other oils, actually help in supporting and cleansing the liver. Hence, ghee is recommended especially when you're sick because the body doesn't need to work to digest it, and it also gives you strength.

For the last couple of months I've been cooking my food in ghee, but it has surprisingly helped stabilize my weight despite my not indulging in a very exhausting yoga routine.

Of course I move around a lot, but I've toned down my vigorous ashtanga routine. Being a yoga teacher, I constantly reinvent my personal practice. But whether I tone it up or down, my weight remains constant when I cook with ghee. This brings me to my next question: is the ghee made from organic, hormone-free cow's milk really the best?

Yes, perhaps it is, especially for therapeutic purposes. However, other types of ghee are not too inferior. In Haryana, where buffalos are prevalent, people eat ghee made from buffalo milk. This milk has more fat. Therefore lesser quantity of buffalo milk (as compared to cow's milk) is required to make the same quantity of ghee. Put simply, we should look at ghee also from a local perspective—the milk of whichever animal is common in the area is best for the people living there.

Here's what I do: I cook with the ghee that we make at home and use the pure, organic cow's milk variety that I buy from a trusted brand to add on top of food or to make medicated ghee. I feel that if we're pouring it on top of food, or using it for medicinal purposes, then the very best quality should be used. If not, don't stress, all ghee is good in my opinion.

Tradition

In India ghee is more than a superfood. It's considered one of the most sattvic (balanced) ingredients and therefore said to enhance the equilibrium of the mind and body. It also has the *prabhava* (special power) to nourish and soothe our cells and tissues. Therefore, it's a great *anupana* (carrier) for any herbal medicine (or even food) as it increases its efficacy. Ghee also has the ability to detoxify the tissues, which is why it's used for *panchakarma* (cleansing) therapies. Cow's milk ghee is supposed to be the most superior for its medicinal effect according to ancient Ayurvedic texts.

When I'd get a sprain or an injury from yoga (which was quite often), I drank 1 tablespoon of ghee with ¼ teaspoon of organic turmeric and a pinch of pepper as suggested by my yoga guru. Because ghee is an excellent carrier, it enhances the healing powers of turmeric and soothes joints and connective tissue. According to Ayurveda, any sort of pain is related to vata, which is responsible for the maintenance of the nervous system. Vata is drying in nature, and ghee, moisturizing. In fact, medicated ghee can deliver better results, especially for joint pains and injuries. There are no painkillers in Ayurveda. However, ghee works on pacifying vata in the joints and turmeric is the best anti-inflammatory, so together they help soothe inflamed, aching tissues.

Ghee also reduces excess *pitta* which shows up as red, inflamed skin and a burning sensation. In fact, the *brajaka pitta* (situated in the skin) gets nourished with the consumption of this wonderful fat. This is how our skin gets moisture and glow just by adding ghee to our diet. When you're consuming medicated ghee in a proper way and at the proper time (see the recipe given later in the chapter) it increases *agni*, which is nothing but appetite, digestion or metabolism. Medicated ghee also crosses the blood–brain barrier, thereby increasing memory and concentration. This is why I consider all forms of ghee to be the basis of any diet that boosts beauty inside and out.

Application

Ghee has a high smoking point (252 degree Celsius), which makes it an ideal cooking medium. As compared to refined, industrial oils that are commonplace in today's kitchens, I believe that ghee is less fattening, and definitely not acidic on the system. While some people say that ghee poured over food (instead of cooking in it) is healthier, I do both. I cook my dals in ghee and then add a little bit extra to enhance the taste of food. I find that more than any other oil or fat, ghee really makes the food taste richer and nuttier. You can drizzle it over lobster, use it to roast vegetables, swirl it into bulletproof coffee instead of butter and add it to popcorn to turn it into a gourmand's delight.

Care must be taken, however, to ensure that ghee is eaten with warm food alone. Do not drink cold drinks or eat cold food with it. Eating it with warm or hot food and drinks ensures that it is digested and assimilated properly. Cold water or drinks with food will congeal the ghee and give you a feeling of indigestion and heaviness.

How to store ghee

Ghee does not go rancid quickly. There are temples which have stored it for even a hundred years. But this type is used for medicinal benefits alone. Just keep it in a clean, dry glass container. However, be careful not to stick a wet or damp spoon in the jar as that may lead to mould.

Ghee is excellent for the body—but if you're not utilizing it; you're just storing it as fat. If you don't have a fitness routine (I strongly encourage that you do), it is best to limit your ghee consumption to about 1 teaspoon a day.

How to Make Ghee at Home

- Collect as much cream as you can (preferably) from organic, hormone-free milk. When you have a substantial amount, transfer the entire contents into a wok and melt on low heat.
- Keep heating for several hours till the milk solids separate and the fat becomes clear with a reddish hue. Then strain the liquid from the sediment into a clean, dry glass jar.

Balancing Medicated Ghee (Ghrita Murchana)

- Take one part ghee, with ¼th part each of coarsely ground triphala, *manjishtha* and haldi powders. Add 16 parts water. Boil it in an iron wok till the water gets fully evaporated. (The reason we use coarse powders is because they're easily strained.)
- Strain and store in a clean glass jar.
- If you want to detoxify your body then eat a teaspoon on an empty stomach every day. To balance all your doshas eat a teaspoon just before breakfast with the first morsel of food.

Note: Do not use a coated wok (non-stick or aluminium) to cook the ghee. In fact, it is best not to use coated vessels at all in cooking because the aluminium and heavy metals get into the food and then our bodies, leading to skin problems. Also, according to Ayurveda, copper and brass must never be used for dairy products.

2

COCONUT

It is the ultimate symbol of joy. Its scent is like a vacation for the mind, its water instantly energizes a tired body and a splash of its milk makes everything tastier. In India, the coconut is revered greatly. We break it open before auspicious occasions as an offering to the gods. It's so purifying, healing and strengthening that it is essential to bless any celebration. The last decade or so has been especially good for the coconut. We have seen a huge surge in its popularity. We're applying the oil to frayed cuticles, split ends, dry skin and even mixing spoonfuls in green tea and coffee. But, as with most natural ingredients that are celebrated, coconut is now being demonized too.

A 2017 research conducted by the American Heart Association found that coconut oil has as much (if not more) fat than butter and even beef fat. And, therefore, the study said that it increases cholesterol and causes weight gain.[1] I don't find it surprising. At the end of the day coconut oil is a saturated fat, and any fat (whether it's saturated or unsaturated) must not be used in excess. The problem arises when we put food up on a pedestal so high that any shortcomings aren't even considered a possibility.

In the last decade or so we have leapfrogged from one food to another, calling each the holy grail of health. There were goji berries, avocadoes, wheat bran, acai, cacao and even red meat, which was part of the Atkins diet. The problem is that the moment a food becomes a fad, we start overusing it without proper knowledge. However, there really is no one superfood that resolves all our problems. All plants and all foods have superpowers—each with its own unique property.

Coconut oil has some wonderful benefits, but too much will, of course, increase cholesterol. And if you consume it with ice cream or a cold drink, it will congeal inside your body because it is a saturated fat just like ghee. But to demonize it to an extent where it's comparable to beef fat is an exaggeration. The one big difference between the two is that beef fat is inflammatory and coconut oil (being plant-based) is anti-inflammatory. Therefore, they're the opposite ends of the spectrum: inflammation causes disease and foods that control it heal our bodies.

Science

What can be said about coconuts that isn't already known? They're rich in trace minerals such as manganese, iron, zinc, copper and selenium, which help in hormone regulation, cell regeneration and even digestion. They also contain small amounts of B vitamins and a ton of fibre, but the real USP is a certain medium-chain fatty acid called lauric acid. When consumed, it turns into monolaurin, which is a strong antimicrobial agent that fights against viral and yeast infections. In addition, coconut oil also contains caprylic acid (a powerful fungus-fighter) and capric acid (a potent yeast killer). Because of these properties it is given to people with poor gut health, as one of the main reasons for that is candida (or yeast) overgrowth.

While a small amount of candida is essential for healthy digestion, in excess it can damage organs and release toxic by-products into the bloodstream. Signs of candida overgrowth include regular migraines, intense sugar cravings, bloating, anxiety, digestive issues and low energy. The three acids mentioned above form a powerful antidote that helps break down candida fungus in the body and restore healthy digestion. A safe amount of coconut oil that you can consume daily is 1 tablespoon. If, however, after a couple of months, you don't see any improvement in your skin, mood or digestion, increase the dosage with the help of a certified nutritionist. Do keep in mind that some of the prime causes for this overgrowth are sugar, wine and antibiotics.

Coconut water is a highly isotonic fluid, meaning the electrolytes in it are very similar to our blood plasma. Therefore it revives us instantly. It's like a hydrating injection, balancing the electrolytes immediately and fortifying the body with amino acids. Coconuts are alkaline in nature and cleansing for the body, which makes their water the perfect drink to kick-start your day.

Coconut meat is high in fibre and therefore helps promote gut health. The MCTs (medium chain triglycerides) in its oil break down as ketones, which serve as fuel for the brain. This is why they're useful for memory problems and improving brainpower.

Tradition

In the Ayurvedic tradition, the coconut tree is called *kalpavriksha*, or a tree that fulfils all wishes. If you think about it, you realize that each and every part of the coconut is useful. It gives us refreshing water and young meat that's packed with vitamins and minerals. The old fruit gives us oil, its outer shell is used to make artefacts, while the husk is used as compost and also stuffed into bedding.

Traditionally we know that mature coconuts (from which the oil is extracted) should be consumed in moderation. But people mostly drink coconut oil that is extracted from the mature fruit. I believe that findings from modern science must be viewed parallelly with the knowledge from our ancestors. In Ayurveda the tender (young) and middle-aged coconuts are considered the best for consumption because they are healing and nourishing for the body. Once the coconut becomes old it's heavy to digest. Old coconut is also heating (ideal for winter), while the young fruit is cooling (perfect for summer). While a mature, hard nut has its benefits, it must be consumed in small quantities. There is also no reference in Ayurveda that suggests that plain oil should be consumed. It's better to cook with coconut oil because it will enhance the quality of food, making it easy for the body to assimilate and digest it.

Coconuts are both sattvic (balanced) and alkaline. Therefore they keep the mind calm and centred. Coconut water is cooling and is a natural diuretic, so it flushes out bacteria and therefore helps to cure urinary infections. The middle-aged coconut in particular builds up all seven *dhatu*s in the body (plasma, blood, muscles, fat, marrow, bone, reproductive fluid).

The primary taste of coconut is sweet, and in Ayurveda this is the most soothing and nourishing taste. Coconuts increase kapha in the body; therefore they can definitely cause weight gain if eaten in excess. However, kapha is also responsible for immunity and strength, and in giving us luminous skin and hair. So they're ideal for those who want to increase their vitality.

Coconut is good for all seasons as it pacifies vata (dryness in winter) and pitta (heat in summer). The only rule is that just like ghee it must be eaten with warm food and drink because it is a saturated fat.

Application

Your diet must consist of 20 per cent fat, which translates into 8–9 teaspoons of oil in a day. From this number, keep 2 teaspoons for coconut oil, and the rest for other fats because more variety will give you a larger range of nutrients.

Coconut oil is said to improve hair quality and strength with its *keshya* properties. It also helps improve the complexion. While most people can apply this oil, some can be allergic to it. This is because it is comedogenic—can clog pores. When I apply and leave it on the skin I get rashes, but it works very well on my hair. Even when I add coconut oil and milk to food, it gives me a sense of nourishment and satiation.

A good way to test it would be to apply the oil on the side of your neck. If, after a few hours, the skin becomes bumpy or red, it's not to be applied. But that doesn't mean that beauty products containing coconut oil will cause a reaction too. The oil is stabilized in cosmetics and therefore works very differently on the skin. Drinking coconut water clarifies the skin—consume it first thing in the morning on an empty stomach, especially during summer.

Coconut-and-Clay Toothpaste

2 teaspoons bentonite clay
1 ½ teaspoons baking soda
½ teaspoon clove powder
½ teaspoon cinnamon powder
2 teaspoons coconut oil
½ teaspoon activated charcoal
A few drops of peppermint oil

- Mix the bentonite clay, baking soda, clove powder and cinnamon powder.
- Add the coconut oil, activated charcoal, a few drops of peppermint oil and a bit of distilled water and mix it all.
- Never use a metal spoon or container to make or store this toothpaste as the negative ions in the bentonite clay will bond with the positive charge in many toxins from metals.
- This amount is enough for two people for a month. Keep it stored in a glass jar and do not use a metal spoon to scoop it out.

- This toothpaste helps clean and whiten the teeth without the harmful toxins (such as fluoride) present in commercial toothpastes.
- Instead of using and throwing plastic tubes, you can also reduce waste by making your own toothpaste.

Mom's Nourishing Coconut Hair Oil

50 ml virgin coconut oil
5–6 fresh red hibiscus flowers or 1 tablespoon hibiscus powder
10–15 curry leaves
2 teaspoons fenugreek seeds
2 teaspoons *brahmi* powder
A fistful of dried amla

- Heat the virgin coconut oil.
- Once the oil is hot, add the hibiscus flowers, curry leaves, fenugreek seeds, brahmi powder and dried amla.
- Let it boil for 2 minutes and switch it off.
- Once cool, store in a glass jar. No need to strain.

This oil improves hair strength, darkens the colour, prevents greying and adds shine.

Amma's Coconut Chutney

1 coconut
½ cup roasted chana dal
2–3 green chillies
1 teaspoon sliced ginger

1 tablespoon coconut or any other cold-pressed cooking oil
½ teaspoon mustard seeds
½ teaspoon chana dal
½ teaspoon broken white lentils (*urad dal*)
10 curry leaves
2 gondu round chillies or whole red chillies
Salt to taste

- Grate a cup of coconut after removing the dark skin.
- Grind it with the roasted chana dal, green chillies, sliced ginger, a cup of water and salt to taste.
- Then heat the oil. When it's hot, add the mustard seeds, chana dal, urad dal, curry leaves and gondu round chillies.
- When it sputters, pour into the paste. Refrigerate till you serve.

Coconut Milk

- Grate 1 coconut (it should give you about 2½–3 cups of grated meat).
- If you're using pre-shredded coconut chips, soak them in warm water for about 2 hours.
- Put the coconut meat, a cinnamon stick (optional) and 1½ cups of water into a blender and blend for about 3–5 minutes.
- Sieve in a cheesecloth or a fine sieve. This is your first press, which is great to make coconut yoghurt, coconut cream and generally to dribble on to a toast.

- Then put the leftover meat into the blender again with 1½ cups of water and blend for about 1–2 minutes.
- Sieve again. This is your second press, which is a great alternative for milk in your smoothies, tea, coffee, turmeric latte or cereal.
- Then put the leftover meat into the blender again with 1 cup of water. Blend for about 30 seconds to 1 minute.
- Sieve again. This is your third press, which can be used in curries, sticky rice or as a salad dressing.

Note: Cinnamon and coconut are a match made in heaven. The former really brings out the latter's natural sweetness. Cinnamon is also a great insulin regulator and this prevents storage of fat and improves metabolism.

3

MUSTARD OIL

I have vivid memories of mustard from my childhood—the pungent taste and smell of the oil, the yellow fields in our village and the sharp taste of mustard saag, softened with dollops of ghee. *Pehelwan*s in traditional *akhada*s use its oil for massages and my grandmother still swears by its rejuvenating properties. But despite being praised for its benefits over the years, this potent oil has gained quite a notorious reputation. Because it contains a high amount of erucic acid (considered toxic in high doses) mustard oil is banned for consumption in the United States.

The most potent healers in the world have poisonous compounds. Look at neem, an insecticide, or bitter apricot oil, which contains amygdalin that's one part cyanide. Indians have been consuming mustard and mustard oil for generations, without any harmful effects. Do you know why? Because we smoke mustard oil before cooking in it, thereby destroying the erucic acid. There's always a reason behind tradition. The way we cook and eat isn't because we follow rituals blindly, but because there is a scientific explanation behind everything. We may not always know the reason, but it's never meaningless.

Science

Mustard belongs to the same family of plants such as cabbage, horseradish (wasabi), turnips and kale, which is why it has a sharp taste like these vegetables. It is high in MUFAs and polyunsaturated fatty acids (PUFAs like omega-3 and omega-6) that are extremely good for the heart. A 2017 study published in the *Journal of Preventive Cardiology* found that using mustard oil as a cooking medium reduced the risk of heart disease by a whopping 70 per cent.[1] Perhaps it's because mustard oil has the ideal 1:2 ratio of omega-6 and omega-3 fatty acids, which is as close as it gets to the recommendations of the World Health Organization for keeping your heart healthy. While omega-3 is anti-inflammatory, omega-6 is pro-inflammatory in excessive amounts. In addition, mustard oil also has low saturated fat as compared to other oils.

Mustard seeds are high in antioxidants, particularly B vitamins and vitamin E. They're also packed with minerals such as calcium, iron, magnesium, manganese, phosphorus, potassium and selenium. These minerals are essential in building bones, cell regeneration, metabolism and water balance, among many other benefits. Even mustard greens have a similar rich nutritional profile and are packed with vitamins A, K, E and C. Perhaps that is the reason why people who consume copious amounts of mustard have beautiful skin and hair. Think of Bengali women who are blessed with radiant skin and thick, dark hair.

As far as the erucic acid controversy goes, there are some animal studies that show a risk of heart disease. However, all the studies have been conducted on mice; there's not a single study that has been conducted on humans. Also, as mentioned earlier, when we smoke mustard oil, we lose the erucic acid in it. These days there are oils with as little as 2 per cent erucic acid but they're genetically modified. When we genetically modify any food, its quality goes down, along with the nutrient content. I like to use organic, cold-pressed oils in their natural form and then use them in the time-tested, traditional manner.

The *kacchi ghani* or cold-press method of extracting the oil ensures that all the components remain intact. The varied essential fatty acids, antioxidants, minerals and the ideal proportion of omega-3 and omega-6, plus the kacchi ghani method of extraction, make mustard oil one of the cheapest and healthiest oils in the world.

Tradition

According to Ayurveda, mustard seeds are heating, pungent, light, dry and penetrating. Because of these qualities they are excellent for pain relief. It's no surprise that wrestlers in akhadas use this oil for massages as it can relieve pain, boost circulation and soothe joints. These properties also make it an excellent hair oil. Massaging your scalp with mustard oil makes hair grow thicker, longer and also prevents it from going grey prematurely. In fact, because it is an anti-inflammatory, a pain reliever, it works very well for gum disease too. Traditionally, in my village, people would massage their teeth and gums with a mixture of mustard oil and salt, instead of toothpaste and toothbrush. They never had a cavity in their lives and also had perfectly formed white teeth.

Mustard has antifungal and antimicrobial effects on the body. When consumed, it helps the body get rid of bad bacteria and fungi like yeast. In Ayurveda it's also recommended for worms and parasites in the body. It's these properties that kill the bad bacteria in the mouth that cause receding, inflamed gums and cavities. Just massaging your gums with a bit of mustard oil can help increase and strengthen tissue in the mouth.

Application

The heating properties of this oil make it excellent for those with weak digestion. Its expectorant (phlegm-inducing) and carminative (sweat-inducing) actions are also good for people with asthma or lung problems. Mustard oil is best for kapha types who suffer from congestion regularly. It also suits vata types who suffer from dry, flaky skin. However you must apply it regularly (at least 3–5 times a week) to get the best results.

The oil is high in vitamin E and works well on both skin and hair. It helps lighten age spots and nourishes the skin. Mustard oil must be massaged well into the scalp and hair to thicken and promote new growth. This helps in reducing itchiness and scalp infections as it destroys all fungi.

One of the lesser-known facts about mustard oil is that it helps reduce plaque. Mix it with a pinch of salt and a few drops of lemon juice and brush your teeth with it daily for four days and see how much cleaner and whiter they look.

This oil is quite heating, so if you are a pitta type it may not be ideal for you. But you can still consume 3–4 teaspoons of mustard oil in a week even if you feel that it may be too heating for you.

4

SATTU

It's ironic but there are some foods off our radar because they're easily available and inexpensive. For some reason health is now an expensive proposition. Or perhaps we expect that we need to pay a lot to be healthy. A case in point are expensive protein powders that we order online, when the solution really lies in our backyards.

Sattu, a flour made of roasted Bengal gram (and sometimes a bit of barley), is available around the corner. It's considered 'poor man's food' as it is popular among those who do manual labour. One of the biggest benefits of this wonderful food is that it makes you immensely robust. Think about it—how do those thin *rickshaw-wallahs* get the strength to pull people double their weight? The answer lies in this genius Indian concoction that was once the staple breakfast in Bihar. There's no reason we cannot go back to the old ways—in fact, we should. Especially because eating sattu for breakfast gives you a boost of protein before you begin the day.

Science

Sattu contains between 15–20 per cent protein by weight. It has both soluble fibres that sweep out cholesterol, along with insoluble fibres that promote healthy elimination. But that's not all. It gives you a massive shot of calcium, magnesium and potassium that together help build strong bones. When you add barley to sattu it gives you manganese that is essential for bone formation. Barley also contains some B vitamins that are essential to make energy from food (B6, 3 and 1), along with minerals including selenium, copper, chromium and phosphorus. However, barley contains gluten, so it must be avoided by those who are allergic or intolerant to it.

These minerals together scavenge free radicals produced by environmental toxins, improve brain function, boost bone health and keep the body cool, among many other benefits. It's no wonder that farmers—who make a meal of sattu—can spend a day working under the harsh Indian sun. Sattu strengthens muscles and bones. When you add a millet like barley and a few nuts it becomes a complete protein. And because the cereals are roasted, and not fried, it contains less than 3 per cent fat.

Tradition

While chickpeas in general are known to increase indigestion, sattū is the opposite because it's made of black Bengal gram (*kala chana*), which is sattvic (centring), easily digestible, non-mucous forming and cooling. Barley too is relatively easily to digest and does not form mucous. Excessive mucous is formed when you have inflammation, and can build up in the throat and chest causing congestion. Anything that reduces excessive immune response, like sattu, will also reduce inflammation and its symptom, phlegm.

Since roasted chana gives you a sense of fullness and satiety, it's recommended during pregnancy to reduce mindless eating. Black gram also purifies the blood and is rich in iron, which gives a rosiness to the complexion.

Application

Sattu is cooling in summer and warming in winter if you add jaggery, dry fruits and spices such as cinnamon. According to Ayurveda, barley is considered very cooling. Therefore it is prudent to switch to plain chana sattu during winter.

Known as the 'poor man's protein', it can be used to make a cooling drink that's highly nutritious. The combination of sattu and jowar (sorghum) may be recommended for those who are recovering from an illness and need to build up their strength. Both are very good sources of protein and fibre and are easily digestible.

Sattu can be made into a shake with soy or almond milk, banana and honey. It can also be made savoury by blending with yoghurt, black salt, coriander and green chillies. During winter, this can be very nourishing and warming. You can make it into a pinni by roasting with ghee, unrefined sugar and all varieties of chopped nuts (see gond laddu recipe).

5

MILLETS

Sunalini is a renowned health editor who is obsessed with millets. She makes millet cakes, uthappams, rotis, porridge and puttu (a Kerala delicacy). Her obsession with these ancestral grains is so strong that her son regularly asks her to bake a normal cake. Did I mention that she is really beautiful and trains for triathlons too?

Millets are older than man himself. They were probably the first grains ever consumed, and in our grandparents' generation, they were staple food. However, in the last few decades, they've been replaced with wheat and rice. In fact, many millets are already on their way to becoming extinct due to lack of consumption.

I became interested in them after I went on an Ayurvedic detox to manage the pain caused by grade IV endometriosis. After replacing wheat with millets I found that I could eat more without feeling bloated or heavy. I also managed to metabolize food better. While earlier I would exercise six days a week to stay in shape, with millets I did not put on weight even when I exercised fewer times a week. I felt lighter and my digestion was much better.

The benefits of millets are numerous. For starters there are so many varieties, with each type offering a different set of vitamins and minerals. They're also hardy grains that grow easily in dry areas, on soil that isn't very fertile and without too much water (they are drought-resistant). This means that (unlike wheat or rice) they require little or no pesticides to grow. They also can be stored for long periods of time because the moisture content of this grain is quite low. At a time when sustainability isn't a luxury but a necessity, millets are the most ecological option available to us.

Eating millets supports small, local farmers who can grow these grains easily without going into debt for seeds, irrigation or pesticides. Ideal for Indian weather, they are local superheroes. Imagine just how low your carbon footprint would be if you started eating grains that came from a village just outside your city? More than anything else, the nutritional content of millets is mind-boggling. I've only explored a few major types, but there are many more varieties, such as foxtail, kodo, proso and little millet available in the market. Try to eat all of them.

Most millets are gluten-free, have a low glycaemic index, are high in fibre and packed with antioxidants, B vitamins and amino acids. Even though they're high in calories they also have a high nutrient-to-calorie ratio, and are therefore not fattening. They're slow to digest and so keep you satiated for long periods, thereby stabilizing your appetite.

However, you must eat these ancient grains according to the season—for instance pearl millet is great for winter and sorghum for summer. Also consume them fresh, preferably in traditional recipes. Packaged food is processed food. Therefore, it is not advisable to eat store-bought millet brownies or chips. As much as possible, eat fresh, eat simple and stay away from 'trending' food.

Barley

One of the earliest cultivated grains, barley is revered for its cleansing and detoxifying properties.

Science

To begin with, it contains more fibre than wheat, rice, amaranth or quinoa. 100 g of barley contains 14 per cent soluble and insoluble fibre to sweep away cholesterol and give bulk to stools so they can be eliminated easily. As we all know, healthy digestion is essential for beautiful skin.

This grain also contains huge amounts of calcium, magnesium, phosphorus and manganese that are required for healthy bones. In addition, it contains vitamin B6 (for healthy nervous system), the important trace mineral selenium (to reduce inflammation and flakiness of skin), iron and folate (to slow down ageing). The beta-glucan fibre present in this millet is the same found in oats and it helps lower blood cholesterol levels. However, it has more protein than oats.

Barley has gluten in it—so if you have a gluten allergy or intolerance stay away from it.

Tradition

In Ayurveda barley is considered cooling and strength-giving. It is traditionally among the grains prescribed in an *ama*-reducing or detox diet. The prescription of barley water for urinary tract infections (UTI) and water retention isn't something new. It has been mentioned as a cure for urine problems even in the *Charaka Samhita*.

Because it's a light, alkaline grain, it reduces inflammation in the body. It cleans the kidneys, reduces blood pressure, cures constipation and makes the skin clearer with its cleansing and detoxifying properties.

Application

Unlike other millets it's relatively easy to roll out rotis with barley, which I feel is the best way to eat it. If you want to use it for detoxification, consume it as an infused water. You can also soak and sprout barley before cooking it lightly and eating it. This reduces the number of anti-nutrients in the grain, making it easy to digest.

Barley Water

- Boil 1 teaspoon of barley in 1½ glasses of water till just a glass is left. Cover and let it sit overnight.

- Strain and drink in the morning on an empty stomach.
- This works especially well if you have recurring UTI.

Exfoliating Body Cleansing Powder

- Mix equal amounts of besan, barley, green gram and fuller's earth, all in powder form. You can make a large batch and keep it stored.
- For dry skin, make a paste with milk or milk cream and honey or aloe vera gel.
- For oily or blemished skin, make a paste with yoghurt or lemon juice diluted with water.
- For mature skin, make a paste with milk cream, honey, aloe vera gel and almond or wheatgerm oil.
- Apply on the face and body. When it begins to dry, remove the pack by scrubbing the skin lightly.
- Wash with lukewarm water followed by a splash of cold water.
- Pat dry and apply moisturizing lotion.
- This is a natural body cleanser that also gently exfoliates the skin.

Bajra

Once a staple food of hardy Indians of the north, bajra or pearl millet has now been replaced with wheat. As children, bajra roti sounded horribly coarse and was something we never wanted to eat. It's only now, when I have a deeper understanding of traditional food, that I've come to appreciate this wonderful millet. Unlike ragi, which is quite dense, the roti from bajra is easier to make and lighter in taste.

Bajra is considered heating for the system, which is why it's avoided in summer. But experts are a bit torn on this. Many feel that we can eat it in summer because we are always in an ultra-cool, air-conditioned environment even during the hottest days. However, I like to follow traditional knowledge and eat according to seasons. Therefore I believe that delicious bajra rotis and khichdi are strictly for winter months.

Science

Bajra is packed with nutrition. It's a great source of protein, with a 100 g offering about 14 per cent protein. It's also an excellent source of iron, along with several other trace minerals such as calcium, magnesium, manganese and phosphorous, all of which are essential for strong bones. Bajra is extremely high in folic acid, B vitamins and zinc, which makes it an ideal food for pregnant women or anyone who wants to improve the quality of their skin and hair.

Tradition

Traditionally bajra is considered to have strength-giving or bodybuilding properties. This is not surprising since it's traditionally a farmer's food. One of its properties, according to Ayurveda, is astringent—a contracting action, which can dry the skin. This is why bajra roti or khichdi is best eaten with a smothering of ghee (or some other fat if you're vegan).

Application

Even though bajra is high in starch it is completely gluten-free. If you have weak digestion it is best to sprout it first, then dry and grind it into a flour. The flour is smooth and can be used to make both rotis and spaghetti.

Nani's Warming Bajra Khichdi

1 big cup whole bajra
2 tablespoons green moong dal
1 teaspoon chana dal
1 tablespoon rice
2–3 tablespoons ghee
Salt to taste

- Take the bajra and pound lightly in a mortar and pestle with a sprinkle of water.
- The peel will separate from the seeds. Toss the seeds to blow away the peel.
- Pound again, this time with a little more force and then toss to separate the peel again. You can even pound and toss it a third time to fully remove the peel from the grains.
- Once the peel is completely removed, coarsely grind it using a mortar and pestle.
- Add the green moong dal, chana dal and rice to the coarsely ground bajra.

- Boil 3 glasses of water. Once it boils, add the bajra mixture by constantly stirring the water to ensure that no lumps are formed. Add salt to taste.
- Cook for about half an hour or till it looks like a porridge.
- Add ghee generously to it and eat.
- You can also skip salt and add sugar to turn it into a porridge that you can eat with (nut or dairy) milk for breakfast.
- This can be kept refrigerated and eaten for up to three days.

Ragi

I love ragi or finger millet not only for its rich, dense almost chocolatey texture but also because among all the grains this has the highest calcium content.

Science

Just a 100 g of ragi has about 350 mg of calcium, plus a variety of amino acids that are essential for healthy skin and hair. The range of amino acids present in ragi (including tryptophan that produces the happy hormone serotonin) makes it an almost complete protein as compared to other grains and cereals.

This millet is one of the few natural sources of vitamin D and is packed with iron too. The red colour of ragi reflects its high antioxidant content. This high-fibre grain has a very low glycaemic index that makes it ideal for people with diabetes. Because it moves slowly through the gastrointestinal tract, it does not make your blood sugar spike suddenly. Low GI foods are also recommended for those who have acne as insulin spikes are often connected to breakouts.

Tradition

Ragi is the staple food of south India. In Ayurveda, it is said to be sweet in taste (therefore nourishing for the tissues) and hot, yet light and dry. Unlike wheat, it's easy to digest, and is also another grain that's part of the traditional Ayurvedic detox.

Application

When you sprout ragi it boosts the content of vitamin C, B vitamins and amino acids. It also has the lowest fat content among all millets. A lot of people compare the taste and density of ragi with chocolate. Roasting the grain makes it darker and nuttier in flavour. I love roasting the whole grain in ghee before making a porridge out of it.

Ragi can cause bloating in some people as it's high in fibre. If you're prone to it, combine this millet with yoghurt, or make a khichdi and add ghee. All millets are drying in nature so they should be consumed with fat.

Express Ragi Breakfast Drink

¼ cup ragi flour
3 cups thin coconut milk
1 tablespoon jaggery powder

- Cook the ragi flour and 2 cups coconut milk in a skillet over medium-to-low heat.
- Stir constantly for 2 minutes, as ragi tends to clump if you don't. When you find the consistency thickening, pour in 1 more cup of coconut milk and simmer for 3 minutes.
- Turn off the gas and add the jaggery powder. This makes 2 cups.
- This is perfect when you're late for work as it cooks fast and you can pour it into a bottle and drink on the go.

Black-Rice-and-Ragi Puttu

⅓ cup ragi
⅓ cup black rice powder (wash black rice, dry in the sun and powder in the mixie)
⅓ cup coconut, divided into 3 parts

- Put the ragi and black rice flour on a plate. Make a well in each mound.
- Pour 10 ml (2 teaspoons) water into each and rub between your fingers to get a wet breadcrumb consistency.
- Take a puttu mould and put in 1 part coconut at the bottom.
- Add the black rice; don't pack it in. Then add another part coconut, followed by the ragi. Top with the last coconut batch. Cover.
- Place a pressure cooker with 2 inches water over the gas and boil the water.

- Cover with a cooker top and place the puttu mould over the hole.
- Steam for 4 minutes. Switch off the gas and keep it in the same position for 2 minutes.
- Take it off the cooker and keep it closed for another 2 minutes. De-mould.
- Enjoy with ghee and shakker (jaggery powder), or a south Indian–style prawn curry.

Ragi Idli

2 cups ragi grains
½ cup *parmal* rice
½ cup idli rice
½ cup urad dal
½ teaspoon fenugreek seeds (*methi dana*)
1 teaspoon salt

- Soak both the rice together in vessel 1, ragi grains in vessel 2 and dal and methi dana together in vessel 3 overnight (12 hours). Soak the grains in triple the quantity of water of the measured quantity of the grain.
- Drain and retain the water of the urad dal. Ensure the dal and water are at the same level in the grinder and start grinding the dal and methi dana. If the batter becomes thick and looks tight, sprinkle some of the retained water a couple of times. It should take about 10 minutes to get a nice and fluffy batter—it should not be very runny. Take out and keep it aside.

- Next, drain the water from the ragi and rice and add it to the grinder. Ensure the ragi and both the rice are at the same level as water in the grinder. Start grinding them together. Add a little more water, if required, to grind the ragi and rice to a smooth and thick batter. This should take about 15–20 minutes.

- Now mix both the urad dal and ragi-and-rice batter well with your hand to aerate it. Keep it covered in a container overnight (12 hours) to let it ferment. The batter should rise up to double its size. Mix it well again using your hand.

- In summer, keep it covered overnight to let the batter ferment without salt and without refrigeration. In winter, add 1 teaspoon salt to the batter and keep it covered overnight without refrigeration.

- Before making the ragi idlis, taste the batter and add salt, if required, in the morning. This also depends on the quantity of idlis being made at the time. Before making it, mix the batter well by hand to aerate it.

- Refrigerate it if you are not making the idlis the same day. Allow the batter to come down to room temperature after taking it out from the fridge. This should take around 15 minutes. Mix well using your hand to aerate the batter.

- In an idli steamer, add 2 cups of water to boil. In the meantime, apply ghee or oil in each mould of the idli plates.

- Pour the batter with a serving spoon into each mould and place it inside the steamer when the water starts boiling. Close the lid and cook for 8–10 minutes.

- Open the lid carefully and insert a thin skewer in the middle of the idli to check if it is cooked. The skewer should come out clean. Turn off the stove.
- Let the idlis cool for few minutes. Scoop them out with a knife or a wet spoon so that they do not crumble.
- Serve hot.

Note: Ragi, rice and dal have to be washed at least 3–4 times before soaking in fresh water. The ratio yields 1.5 kg of batter to make 20–22 idlis or 15 dosas.

Jowar

Drought-tolerant and heat-resistant, this hardy grain, also known as sorghum, is another delicious farmer food. In Haryana, where once women used to work in the fields, bajra and jowar were the staple carbohydrates.

Science

Like other millets, sorghum is also rich in fibre and B vitamins, along with bone-builders such as calcium, magnesium and phosphorus. Just a single serving of jowar provides you with more than 50 per cent of your required daily allowance of copper, which increases the absorption of iron and prevents premature ageing. Its colour—ranging from light to dark brown—reflects its high antioxidant content, which protects you from environmental pollution. The waxy matter around the grain contains substances called policosanols that are known to reduce cholesterol in the body.

Tradition

While sorghum isn't as strengthening as bajra, it is traditionally considered extremely cooling and therefore should be consumed in the summer. When my grandmother was young, and sorghum was freely grown in the farms, they would eat the green seeds raw or boiled in water. Unfortunately, jowar, like many other millets, is rarely grown now and is hard to find in its fresh, green form.

Application

You can eat this grain all year, use it as a gluten-free replacement for cakes or just pop and add it as a crunchy element to salads. I find that sorghum flour is especially crumbly so it's very difficult to make rotis with it. To make the flour malleable, you can add a bit of rice flour and boiled potato. Or you can just make it sprout and add it to salads.

Millet Breakfast Brownies

6 eggs
3 small cups jaggery powder
1½ small cups organic coconut oil
1 small cup organic raw cacao powder

1 small cup jowar
1 small cup ragi
¼ teaspoon baking soda
A handful of flax seeds
1 small cup mixed dry fruits, finely chopped (you can also use 2 types of raisins)

- Separate the egg whites and yolks.
- Beat the egg whites with an electric mixer until they start looking like firm cream.
- Add the jaggery powder and beat for 2 more minutes.
- Add the egg yolks and beat for some time.
- Now mix in the rest of the ingredients gently with a spoon: First, gently stir in the cacao and coconut oil. Once the batter is smooth, add the millets mixed with baking soda. Add the flax seeds and dry fruits last.
- Preheat the oven to 220 degrees Celsius for 3 minutes.
- Pour the batter into a 9.5-inch non-stick baking pan (oil the pan before pouring it).
- Bake for 20 minutes on 200 degrees Celsius. Poke with a fork to see if the brownies are completely baked (if they are, nothing should stick).
- Cut and serve.

6

RICE

Rice is the ultimate comfort food. It's light, easily available and, of course, delicious. I grew up with wheat as my staple food—rice was a rare treat. We had it perhaps only a couple of times in a month. I didn't know then that wheat didn't suit me. Because the pesticide-laden, genetically modified wheat varieties available after the 1970s were highly inflammatory, my skin was always red and bumpy.

Then, a few years ago, I drastically reduced my wheat consumption to keep endometriosis under control. Brown rice became my staple carb and soon, because of this switch, my skin finally started looking smooth and even-toned. Even refined white basmati rice worked better for me than wheat. I know of dermatologists who look ten years younger than their actual age who survive on rice.

Science

Polished white rice has its downsides. Because its husk has been removed, it has a high glycaemic index, which means that it gets digested quickly, transforming into sugar and raising insulin levels. It is important to keep portion control in mind while consuming rice in general, whether it's white, brown, red or black rice. We should treat it as one of the elements on the plate and not as the main dish. So take equal quantities of lentils, vegetables and rice. Also, if you're eating polished white rice, combine it with vegetables, lentils and yoghurt. The fibre in the vegetables and lentils lowers the glycaemic index of the entire meal. Rice also contains the amino acid missing in lentils. Therefore, our traditional combination of dal and chawal is actually a complete protein.

You can also opt for high-fibre and nutrient-rich varieties such as brown, red and black rice. Packed with fibre, B vitamins and minerals, just a cup of cooked brown rice provides you 88 per cent of your required daily amount of manganese, a mineral that supports bone health and prevents the onset of osteoporosis. It also contains the trace mineral selenium, a powerful antioxidant, along with magnesium and phosphorus that are essential for strong bones. Add to that a good amount of B6 that promotes healthy skin (among many other benefits) and you have a 'superfood' that is probably already in your kitchen. Because of its rich fibre content brown rice is an effective tool against heart disease because the fibre binds with the cholesterol to pull it out of the body.

Sadly, rice has faced the same destiny as wheat. From more than a lakh indigenous varieties, the number has come down to less than 6000 today. How many of them are actually available to us? When we eat indigenous grains we're eating the food meant for us according to our genetics and geographic location. When we eat locally, we eat in harmony with the land, the seasons and our own body types. Eating a wide variety of each ingredient and food in general gives us that many more nutrients. If there are any rules of beauty food I'd say it would be these three—eat local, seasonal and also a wide variety of foods. Because rice is such a staple, it's even more essential to rotate its variants so that with each spoonful we get more nutrition.

Tradition

Ayurveda considers unpolished, long-grain basmati rice superior to other varieties. In both taste and post-digestive affect (called *vipaka*), basmati is sweet. This means that it is comforting, strengthening and nourishing for the tissues. It has a cooling effect on the body and is a purely sattvic food that helps balance all the doshas. However, unpolished basmati is recommended over the polished variety.

Application

Traditionally, it is recommended that rice must be cooked in a copper vessel to enhance all its properties. Copper is an essential trace mineral that is responsible for collagen production; therefore cooking in a vessel made with this metal makes rice a beauty food. You can also add one or two pinches of cumin seeds and two or three black peppercorns to rice while cooking so it becomes light and easy to digest. According to Ayurveda it is best to begin your meal with something sweet. It cuts down your appetite and tendency to binge by half. Therefore, a small quantity of rice mixed with ghee and unrefined sugar (*khand*) can be eaten first. This sweet rice treat is also considered immensely moisturizing and nourishing for the entire body. However, you must never drink anything cold with your meals as the ghee will congeal and feel heavy in your body.

How to Cook Rice for Nutrition

While most people tend to drain the water after cooking rice, by doing so you are throwing away the amino acids. You should cook rice in a way that the water gets fully absorbed into the grain and it holds on to its nutrients. The water from boiled rice is considered so nutritious that often just the liquid is recommended for people with poor appetite or those recovering from an illness. Even women who have menstrual problems are given Ayurvedic medicine along with this water.

How to Cook Rice for Weight Loss

Rice should be soaked for at least an hour so that the enzymes present in them become easier to digest. It also leeches out any harmful chemicals through the process of osmosis. Another way to cook rice is to add a spoonful of coconut oil in the water while it is boiling. The oil mixes with the starch in the rice and alters the composition of the starch molecules. After the rice is cooked and the extra water drained, it should be chilled. This creates resistant starches (starches that resist digestion) that the body uses as fibre rather than carbs. This stays even after the rice is reheated before consumption.

Brown Rice Dosa

1 cup unpolished brown rice
¼ cup broken urad dal
¼ cup chana dal
½ teaspoon methi dana
¼ teaspoon asafoetida (*hing*)
1 teaspoon salt

- Soak all the first 4 ingredients in water overnight. Soak the grains in triple the quantity of water of the measured quantity of the grains.
- Drain and retain the water of the soaked ingredients. Ensure the ingredients and water are at the same level in the grinder and start grinding it all together. If the batter becomes thick and looks tight, sprinkle a little of the retained water a couple of times. It should take about 18–20 minutes to get a nice and fluffy batter. The batter should not be very runny. Take it out and keep aside.
- Add ¼ teaspoon hing and mix the batter. Keep it covered in a container overnight (12 hours) to let it ferment. The batter should rise up to double its size. Mix it well again using your hand after fermentation.
- In summer, keep it covered overnight to let the batter ferment without salt and without refrigeration. Before making the dosas, taste the batter and add salt, if required, in the morning. This depends on the quantity of dosas being made. Before making the dosas, mix the batter well by hand to aerate it.

- In winter, add 1 teaspoon salt to the batter. Keep it covered overnight to let the batter ferment without refrigeration. Before making the dosas, taste the batter and add salt, if required, in the morning. This depends on the quantity of dosas being made that time. Before making the dosas, mix the batter well by hand to aerate it.
- Spread the batter on a non-stick tawa. Add a mixture of oil and ghee on the edges of the dosa to make it crisp. As it becomes crisp, roll it.
- You can eat it with coconut and tomato chutney.

Other Varieties

Red Rice

Red rice is similar to brown rice except that its colour comes from the presence of anthocyanins, antioxidants usually found in red or purple fruits and vegetables. It also contains huge amounts of fibre and has the same nutritional profile as the brown variety. The traditional red rice that comes from south India is considered to be the best according to Ayurveda. Called *rakthashali*, it is said to be nutritious and medicinal. Ancient texts suggest that this variety of rice helps improve eyesight, works as a diuretic and has a cooling, antitoxic effect on the body.

Black Rice

Did you know that just a spoonful of black rice bran contains more antioxidants than a spoonful of blueberries? And that too with much more fibre and far less sugar. It also contains vitamin E, another powerful antioxidant, along with iron. The high fibre and antioxidant content of black rice makes it a good ally against heart disease and, of course, without doubt helps boost the health of skin and hair too. Also, the phytonutrient mix in black rice helps the liver remove unwanted toxins from the body.

For me, black rice is a real treat. It has an almost berry-like aftertaste because of which it is a popular base for dessert. It is one of those rare foods that tastes decadent, is high in nutrition and low in calories.

Black Rice Glow Bowl

¼ cup cooked black rice
½ mango, chopped
1 cup thick coconut milk
2 tablespoons condensed milk or 2 minced prunes or dates (optional)

- Assemble all the ingredients.
- Mix and eat.

7

RAW HONEY

Warming, nourishing and cleansing, honey is the ultimate beauty food—whether you eat or apply it. Unfortunately, honey finds itself in the midst of the current war against sugar. Of course refined sugar is bad. However, I do believe that sweetness is an essential taste and sugars such as honey and jaggery, when consumed in small quantities, are actually good for you.

I've always considered honey a nectar of health. Unlike refined sugar that's acidic, it has an alkaline effect on the body. When our body is acidic, there is increased inflammation, which eventually leads to disease. Alkalinity, on the other hand, is calming, pacifying and disease-fighting. Honey is a gift from nature—it's delicious to eat and even more wonderful to apply as a mask or a cleanser. When it comes to beauty it has to be the most basic addition to your cabinet.

Science

Delicious and nourishing as honey may be, it's probably one of the most contaminated foods in the market. Most of the varieties available are overheated, liquefied, diluted and pasteurized. Heating and pasteurization removes the precious enzymes and antioxidants that make it such a potent healer. When diluted and over-processed, honey loses its medicinal value and is just like refined sugar. However, raw, unpasteurized honey contains more than twenty amino acids and about 5000 enzymes. It also contains trace amounts of B vitamins, along with iron, zinc, potassium and calcium. One of the main enzymes in honey is called amylase, which helps breaks down carbs like potatoes or bread. The other enzymes in this nectar help in the digestion and assimilation of food.

All types of raw honey have antibacterial qualities, however the action varies, depending on the beekeeper's ability, environmental conditions and the botanical origin of the nectar. Manuka honey, for instance, is considered extremely precious because the bees feed on the flowers of the manuka plant. I've used manuka essential oil—it's so potent that just a drop of the essential oil in your face cleanser helps clarify the complexion. Therefore manuka honey is bound to be medicinal.

Raw honey contains many antioxidants and phenolic compounds that it gets from plants. This high antioxidant content has beneficial effects on cardiovascular health as it reduces inflammation and protects the heart from oxidative stress. Because of this reason, it is beneficial for the skin and hair. It also contains hydrogen peroxide, a natural antiseptic that eliminates bacteria and fungus, and thus improves the complexion on application.

Tradition

In Ayurveda, honey is nourishing, heating, energizing and detoxifying. Its emetic (phlegm-clearing) and soothing properties make it excellent for coughs and cold. It is said that even taking honey steam is beneficial and can provide instant relief for asthma patients. Honey is easy to digest and helps in detoxifying the colon of waste matter. Its antibacterial or antifungal properties also make it a boon for oral health. You can massage honey on your gums and teeth to prevent decay, or gargle with honey water to soothe inflammation of the throat.

Honey is beneficial for healing wounds and can be applied on irritated skin. It is also part of the Ayurvedic *varnya* category of ingredients that is supposed to clarify and brighten the complexion. It is considered to be so good for the eyes that in some Ayurvedic treatments it is applied inside the socket (don't try this at home, kids!). Because it pacifies pitta and kapha it is good for the skin and helps with obesity. Honey with warm water is recommended for those who want to reduce weight. It has scraping qualities; therefore it cuts down fat in the body, though in limited quantities.

Honey is also an excellent catalyst that increases the effect of any herbs or medicine that is given along with it. Its hot, penetrating quality ensures that the effect of any treatment goes right to the cellular level, making herbal medicine more bioavailable for the body. Because of its heating and energizing properties, it also works as a tonic in old age.

Application

Organic, raw honey is my favourite base for a face mask. Most people like to use milk, cream or water, but I love honey. Because it has anti-inflammatory qualities, honey can reduce symptoms of rosacea. I definitely find my skin looking clearer after its application. Even if I don't have anything else I mix an egg white in it to apply all over my face. It's a great pre-party fix because it makes the skin look more toned and clear. You can even make an everyday exfoliator with honey—just mix raw honey and powdered rolled oats and use it every day to wash your face. Both honey and oats are calming and soothing for red, inflamed complexions and so this combination works like a balm for sensitized skin.

Honey is also a great humectant, i.e., it attracts moisture. If your skin is oily and acne-prone, and you've assaulted it with harsh, drying treatments, honey will soothe your skin and take away the dryness, but without making it oily. It contains antioxidants to protect the complexion and enzymes to increase cell turnover. Plus, it works as an antibacterial agent to keep breakouts at bay.

For dry skin too honey is a great healer, especially because of its moisturizing properties. I like to 'loosen' honey with a bit of rosewater, add a couple of drops of my favourite face oil and then use it as a base for a face mask when my skin is dry. The best part is that when we use honey in masks they take much longer to dry, keeping the healing ingredients (whatever is in your mask) on your face for longer.

While honey is great for application, its internal benefits are even more astounding. Being a great catalyst it increases the effect of any herb that is consumed along with it. One very effective and safe combination to boost immunity and get rid of skin conditions such as eczema and psoriasis is 1 teaspoon each of giloi powder and honey. The former is the best immune modulator, which is why it is effective in autoimmune conditions such as psoriasis. The latter is a pitta pacifier, so it gets rid of burning sensations. Take it on an empty stomach for at least six months to see results. For therapeutic purposes the honey should be at least a year old.

Honey is also a time-tested remedy for cough. Take 1½ tablespoons of ginger juice with 1 teaspoon of honey 15 minutes before lunch and dinner to increase your appetite and soothe the throat. You can also take 1 teaspoon each of fresh tulsi juice and honey if you have a cough.

While this nectar has myriad benefits, anything more than 2–3 teaspoons a day can cause drowsiness and intoxication—almost like a hangover. You should never mix honey with anything hot (including hot water), fish, meat or ghee. Old Ayurvedic texts say that equal parts of ghee and honey mixed together work like poison. It's also prudent to consume very small amounts of honey during summer.

Pure honey must never be heated. It must be kept at room temperature and should be eaten on its own or as a carrier for herbs. It becomes toxic over 42 degrees Celsius; its properties change and it becomes indigestible. Therefore it's best to not bake or cook with raw honey. While it is safe for everyone to use, it must not be consumed if you have digestive issues.

The honey purity test

Pure, raw honey should be thick and viscous. If you drop it in a glass of room-temperature water, it should drop right to the bottom without dissolving immediately. When dropped on a paper or cloth, it should not be absorbed by it. When poured on your thumb, it will stay at one place and not run down. Also, pure honey is flammable. When a wick is dipped, it lights up exactly like wax. Adulterated honey, on the other hand, will not light up because it has a high moisture content.

Oatmeal-and-Honey Face Scrub

2 tablespoons raw oatmeal
1 tablespoon honey
½ teaspoon almond oil
2 tablespoons milk
2 tablespoons yoghurt

- Mix all the ingredients to make a coarse paste.
- Apply it all over the face and neck. Leave it for 10–15 minutes. Then wash off and pat dry.
- Oatmeal, milk and honey moisturize and soothe the skin and prevent acne. Yoghurt and oil boost moisture levels, but if your skin is breakout-prone you can leave out the oil. You can use this scrub 1–2 times a week, but do not use it on active breakouts or acne.

8

JAGGERY (GUR)

As children, my brother and I were never allowed any sweets except small pieces of *gur*. We called it black toffee because of its dark red colour and rich taste. During those days, when television was rare, our favourite activity was to tiptoe into the kitchen and grab fistfuls of gur and *churan* while our mother slept in the afternoon. All through our summer holidays we'd eat almost a dozen nuggets everyday—mostly out of boredom but also because stealing them was quite an expedition. You see, our mother is a light sleeper and would get massively irritated if she were disturbed.

Despite eating large quantities of jaggery, my brother and I haven't had a single cavity till today. I think it has a lot to do with the farmer's food we ate (rotis, vegetables, milk, lots of ghee) and, of course, eating gur instead of commercial sweets.

Science

Jaggery has seen a recent surge in popularity because refined sugar has replaced fat as the health enemy number one. So we're stirring it into beverages, adding it to kheer and even using it to make banoffee pie. These days it is even more popular because it is the one ingredient that is said to detoxify your body from air pollutants. However, there is nothing in Ayurvedic texts or science that directly backs up this claim. It clears mucous, soothes the respiratory system and also works against allergies, so perhaps it helps in an indirect manner. Jaggery is sugar but it's not empty calories. With iron, magnesium, potassium and manganese, it has all the minerals that bestow the body with strength and energy.

Tradition

Made from sugarcane, jaggery is considered heating, detoxifying and strengthening. It may not contain a lot of fibre but it helps in digestion by encouraging peristaltic movement (alternate contraction and relaxation) of the colon and intestines. Even in Ayurveda it is recommended for coughs and colds. Its warming properties make it a nourishing tonic for the joints, especially during winter. It purifies the blood, cleans the bladder, increases bulk in stools, boosts the haemoglobin count and builds immunity. In traditional medicine, jaggery that is more than a year old is considered to have medicinal properties and is revered as a cardiac tonic. But it should not be more than three years old. Fresh jaggery is also good but it should be reddish brown in colour and not yellow as the latter could be weaker in potency or contaminated. The red variety is what works best for kapha or the tendency towards congestion, cough and cold.

Application

My evening snack is a small piece of jaggery with roasted black Bengal gram (chana). It is the most delicious and nourishing snack that is high in protein, yet low in calories. I also like to crumble jaggery over a crispy roti with ghee and eat it like a dessert.

If you want to improve strength and immunity, it's best to have a small piece with a cup of warm milk in the morning. This is a wonderful Ayurvedic combination because milk has everything except iron, which you can get from gur. Jaggery also contains potassium, so with milk it is especially good for women as it strengthens bones and increases the haemoglobin levels. If, however, you are lactose-intolerant, you may combine it with a nut milk. Do keep in mind that this is not a traditional combination.

It's important to keep in mind that jaggery is sugar. So if you're not exercising, too much of it will make you put on weight. But I don't believe in cutting out a food group; everything has to be consumed in small quantities. Sweet is also one of the six tastes in Ayurveda. While many of you may argue that one can eat sweet fruits, they're hardly as satisfying as a piece of gur or a spoonful of honey.

Jaggery is best suited for winter because it is warming in nature. A small piece can be eaten after meals for better digestion. However, it is best consumed with milk or tea. Also, according to Ayurveda, it should not be eaten with radish or fish. You can add it to puddings but only after they have cooled down a little because it can curdle milk.

The jaggery purity test

Good-quality jaggery must be sweet, hard and dark brown in colour. It should not be salty (a sign that it's too old) or bitter, nor should it leave a sandy residue in the mouth.

Jaggery Vermicelli

1 cup vermicelli
2–3 tablespoons crumbled jaggery
2 tablespoons ghee

- Boil the vermicelli (brown rice vermicelli if you want it to be healthy). Strain it and then add ghee and crumbled jaggery on top.
- Eat when hot so that the ghee doesn't congeal.

Winter Jaggery Snack

1 cup roasted peanuts
2–3 tablespoons shakker (powdered jaggery)
2–3 tablespoons ghee

- Roughly hand-crush some roasted peanuts. Add powdered jaggery to this, followed by some ghee.
- Serve it as an accompaniment to any Indian winter meal.

9

ASHWAGANDHA

Until recently ashwagandha was thought to be only for men—to enhance their sexual prowess. But this powerful shrub is so much more than just an aphrodisiac. It's a miraculous adaptogen, meaning that it helps your body cope with the effects of stress. It helps reduce fatigue, boosts energy levels, improves the cognitive function of the brain and enhances memory.

Everything that you eat affects your mind and body in equal measure, but ashwagandha in particular builds endurance not just for the body but also for the nervous system. This has made it hugely popular, especially in today's age when stress has emerged as the main catalyst for physical and mental diseases. I like to take an Ayurvedic jam that looks similar to chyawanprash called *ashwagandhadi lehyam*. It's a vegetarian preparation with cumin and liquorice in it. For the last couple of months I have been pushing myself too hard. Other than devoting time to my book, I have also been developing my blog, writing for many publications and teaching and practising yoga on a regular basis. This jam gives me that extra boost of energy when I feel depleted.

Science

One of the main reasons this herb works so well on stressed individuals is because it reduces the level of cortisol, the stress hormone. When we're under immense pressure our body goes into a fight or flight mode. This protective mechanism is built into our systems to help us fight against or flee away from a dangerous situation. When we feel stressed or cornered, the body produces glucose that gives us the energy to fight or run away from a situation. But repeated stress, a hallmark of modern living, leads to constantly elevated glucose levels, leading to many lifestyle diseases.

Stress is the cause behind many modern ailments such as increased blood sugar, blood pressure, inflammation and lowered immunity. A study published in *The Indian Journal of Psychological Medicine* in 2012 showed that ashwagandha substantially reduces the cortisol levels in the body.[1] But that's not all. This herb also helps repair damaged neurons and strengthens the nervous system. It's so powerful that doctors also prescribe it to help improve symptoms of neurodegenerative diseases such as Parkinson's and Alzheimer's.

Since it strengthens the nerves and reduces cortisol levels, ashwagandha has a calming effect on the mind. It has also been found to work as a mood stabilizer for people suffering from anxiety and depression. Studies have shown that ashwagandha enhances mental and physical stamina and boosts sports performance. In an eight-week study, forty elite Indian cyclists (those who have participated in at least state-level tournaments) were divided into experimental and placebo groups. The experimentalists were given 500 mg of ashwagandha roots every day. After eight weeks of supplementation, tests showed that there was a significant improvement in the health of the people belonging to this group. Experimentalists showed a boost in all parameters such as oxygen utilization and consumption and time to exhaustion on the treadmill as compared to the placebo group, which didn't show any change.[2]

Ashwagandha also has anti-carcinogen and anti-tumour properties, which is why it is recommended as an alternative therapy for people who have cancer. This wonderful herb has also shown promise in providing pain relief, especially in chronic, inflammatory conditions such as arthritis and cervical spondylosis. However, it must be kept in mind that no herb is a panacea for health. Your lifestyle, diet, sleep, exercise and mindset all contribute to a reduced tendency towards disease.

Tradition

Traditionally, ashwagandha falls under the group of herbs that bestow the body with strength, nourishment and immunity. Hot in potency, it is considered a *rasayana*, an anti-ageing elixir. It builds muscle, makes wounds heal faster, helps relieve itching and brings down inflammation. These properties make it a great addition to face oils, mists and masks too. In Ayurveda it is useful in vata disorders that are neurological in nature. An interesting fact about this herb is that while it boosts energy and stamina, it also helps in sleep disorders, working as a mild sedative.

Application

It's best to take ashwagandha in a *churna* or powder form instead of a capsule. The ideal quantity is 3–6 g or 1 teaspoon with a cup of milk once a day. According to Ayurveda, ashwagandha is hot, bitter and pungent, while milk is sweet and calming. People with delicate stomachs may find it too hot, so the addition of milk is required to balance its potency. You can also take it with ghee or in a traditional form like the ashwagandhadi lehyam. Ashwagandha, like amla, is a major component of chyawanprash, which is perhaps one reason why it has such strengthening and immune-boosting properties.

Animal fat is the best anupana or carrier of ashwagandha. If you are very weak and emaciated, have it with a cup of bone soup. If you want to improve sleep, take it with buffalo milk. To improve immunity, take it with cow milk. Consume it with ghee if you feel weak or dizzy to nourish tissues and improve nerve strength. If you're vegan, you can take it with hot water. Consume it first thing in the morning on an empty stomach with one of these combinations and then eat breakfast after 30–45 minutes. Eating it in the powder form is better than popping a capsule as the latter can cause abdominal discomfort and bloating.

If you're taking the ashwagandhadi lehyam, have 1 teaspoon twice a day with warm milk or hot water. The jam is more delicious than the powder, and contains other ingredients, so the effect is more fortifying for the entire body. Take it first thing in the morning and then 30–45 minutes before dinner. A lot of people mix ashwagandha into smoothies—while that will not harm you, it will not give you as many benefits as taking it in the traditional manner.

If you have digestive issues or a lack of appetite, you should not take ashwagandha. This is because it is hot in nature and can make abdominal discomfort worse. And when your appetite is lacking, your body will not be able to absorb its benefits completely. Discontinue its use if you experience palpitations, nausea or headaches. If you're taking any medicines for blood pressure, depression or nervous disorders, consult a doctor. Remember to also avoid drinking too much coffee or alcohol with this herb.

Ashwagandha must be taken regularly for a long term (at least six months) for it to have an effect. Any herbal formulation slowly changes your body when taken regularly. Unlike allopathic medicine that shows immediate effect but causes long-term side effects, herbs heal when they're taken with discipline and regularity. When had over a period of time, they truly transform the body, without causing any harm.

10

MUNAKKA

My *nani* always says that if you put a few drops of water from a soaked *munakka* (dried large grape) into the mouth of a dying person, he or she would come back to life. She begins her day with soaked munakkas and so do I when I need that extra boost of energy. Unlike *kismis*, which is small, seedless and golden or green in colour, munakka is much larger and darker and comes with a seed. Its chewy consistency makes it a tasty and healthy dessert—it's one of the few health foods that offer great flavour too.

Science

Raisins and currants are one of the best sources of flavonoids, which are powerful antioxidants that protect us from environmental toxins. They contain fibre, protein, small amounts of minerals such as iron and calcium and B vitamins. They are also abundant in a flavonoid called catechin. Catechins prevent cell damage and fight disease. This makes catechin-rich foods such as green tea, red wine, dark chocolate and our humble munakkas powerful tools to fight age-related wear and tear.

Tradition

Grape is considered the best fruit in Ayurveda. Its cooling quality calms the mind, especially when you're feeling frazzled or tired. It works as a mild laxative, soothes acidity and also reduces the effects of alcohol on the body.

Munakkas have been traditionally used to cure anaemia, give strength to the body and impart a healthy glow. They're recommended for people recovering from mental or physical trauma, or an illness. If you're low on energy, snack on these. Because they are diuretic, they help improve the health of kidneys too. According to Ayurveda, munakkas help build all the tissues in the body, especially the muscle. If you're extremely thin with a dull, dry complexion, eating them for six months will bring you back to a healthy weight and make your skin look luminous. What more can you ask for?

Application

These giant raisins must always be soaked and then consumed on an empty stomach in the morning. If you're an athlete, you can have a whole fistful before a game to energize yourself. When I used to practise ashtanga yoga, I would eat munakkas before my class. Though yoga should be practised on a relatively empty stomach, I could eat them as they were light and provided me with energy.

If you're anaemic, you can have munakkas after soaking them in milk. Drop 10–15 pieces in a cup of hot (nut or dairy) milk. Let them soak for 10 minutes. Then eat the raisins and drink the milk. This concoction is considered highly beneficial for old people or those recovering from an illness. At home we soak munakkas in water overnight. In the morning we drink the water and eat the soaked raisins. It works as a laxative, energizer and nourisher especially when combined with soaked almonds and walnuts. Consuming them in this way also helps soothe pitta conditions.

Fun fact

Eating fresh grapes when you're drinking helps reduce the effects of alcohol. Because they fill you up you'll be less tempted to go for that extra glass of wine and wouldn't want to eat junk food either.

These days I take about 10–15 soaked munakkas and almonds each morning. While I do believe that we must go beyond taste and eat some unappetising food for health, there's nothing like beginning your day on a delicious note. The great thing about munakka is that there are so many ways of consuming them. And each with a different effect. The Western world hasn't caught on to these as much, but here in India, especially in our grandparents' generation, this was the standard energizing health food.

11

TRAGACANTH GUM (GOND)

While I've found that being wheat-free suits me best, come winter, I make an exception for the delicious, crackling *gond* laddus. Made with ghee-roasted gram, wholewheat flour, an assortment of dry fruits and crispy, crunchy gond, this laddu is the ultimate strengthener. We only eat it in winter because it is believed that gond, when roasted, warms the body. In the modern day, we would call this traditional laddu an energy ball. But while energy balls (made with cacao, chia seeds, dates and nuts) work very well as an on-the-go snack, gond laddus are an entire meal in themselves. Think about it—they have whole grains, ghee, nuts and a potent food like gond.

Lovneet Batra, who is a nutrition consultant for this book, told me an interesting anecdote from her childhood. When she was small she couldn't eat mangoes because they'd make her nose bleed. It was only when her mother gave her a glass of Roohafza mixed with gond that she could eat the mangoes. When mixed in water this gum is cooling, and when roasted in ghee it is warming. She reckons that not only was it cooling but it also strengthened the tissues, preventing her nose from bleeding.

Science

Gond is fortified with protein, calcium and magnesium, so it basically builds both muscle and bone. It also comes with a wide variety of amino acids that are essential for healthy skin and hair. Due to its high fibre content, this gum helps in cardiovascular disease, diabetes and digestive problems. Gond also works as a prebiotic, meaning it serves as food for the healthy bacteria in your gut. What's more, it is very soothing for your stomach and improves your gut barrier by increasing bacteria that produce butyrate, which nourishes and builds up the cells in the intestinal wall. Because of all these reasons, gond fortifies, detoxifies, strengthens and boosts immunity.

Tradition

Traditionally, this gum is revered for its many medicinal benefits. It speeds up the healing of wounds, soothes burns, helps in dental problems, improves digestion, reduces bloating, aids in maintaining a healthy body weight and also acts as a blood purifier. Eating small quantities of gond that has been fried in ghee increases the strength of the body, clears cough, opens up the chest and protects the lungs. When it comes to increasing vitality, ghee and gond are a wonderful combination. Together they nourish the joints and connective tissue, ensuring that you have flexibility and no pain in the joints as you grow older. It is no wonder then that gond is recommended by Ayurveda for inflammatory conditions such as rheumatic arthritis. It soothes, nourishes and builds up tissue and gives warmth to the body in the cold months of winter.

Application

Gond is used in laddus, in cooling summer sherbets and even as a thickener in soups. However, if your intestinal system isn't too strong, you may not be able to digest it. It is essential to drink a lot of water when eating this gum so that it moves through your gastrointestinal tract easily.

Gluten-Free Gond Laddu

3 cups besan (chickpea) or sattu flour
¾ cup gond
2 cups ghee
1 ½ cups almonds
1 cup cashew nuts
1 cup dried figs soaked in water and then squeezed out, chopped
1 cup dry dates, soaked and chopped
1 tablespoon poppy seeds
¼ cup unsalted green pistachio
1 cup raisins
1 ½ cups grated dry coconut
2 cups grated jaggery or jaggery powder
1 teaspoon nutmeg powder
1 teaspoon cardamom powder

- Remove the seeds from the dry dates and roast them on low heat. Let them cool down.
- Powder the roasted dates in a mixer.
- Heat 2 tablespoons of ghee and add the gond and fry it until it becomes crispy. When you break it, it should not be sticky inside. Keep aside.
- Grind the gond and coconut into a powder.
- Roast the besan on medium-to-low heat until it becomes very light and its colour changes. A nice aroma will start coming out of it.
- Now add 2 cups of ghee to the roasted flour. Stir it for another 4–5 minutes on medium-to-low heat.
- Add the roasted coconut and gond powder to it and stir it for 2–3 minutes.
- Add the dry fruits, poppy seeds and dry dates powder to it and mix it nicely.
- Add the grated jaggery, cardamom powder and nutmeg powder and remove from the heat.
- Mix well until the jaggery is mixed properly. Roll into laddus.

Note: Clean the dry dates, dried figs, raisins, almonds, pistachios and cashew nuts by rubbing them with a clean towel.

Summer Gond Cooler

2 teaspoons gond
2 tablespoons khus syrup
4 cups (nut or dairy) milk

- Soak the gond in water till it swells to more than double its size.
- In a glass, layer the soaked gond with the khus syrup and milk.
- Serve immediately topped with some ice cubes.

~

'Your body is a beautifully designed machine, so capable of healing itself. When it gives you pain or discomfort, it is sending you a message about what is going on inside. Food is the real medicine. It gets to the root of the problem by supporting your natural ability to heal. True beauty is then a very natural expression of inner vitality and good health. But it goes beyond that. What stupidity it is to limit the definition of beauty to how your features are placed. Being pretty is just appearance. Inner strength and a connection to purpose—now those are real assets. To own who you really are, to take care of your body, to look outside of yourself and serve others with energy and grace, that for me is beautiful.'

—Bharat Mitra, founder, Organic India

~

PART II
CLARITY

Angry, inflamed skin is a sign of inner conflict. It is a reflection of the fight that our bodies put up against impurities that are part pollution, part the foods we eat and part the thoughts we choose. We know now that there is a connection between our habits, mood and the clarity of skin. One leads to another. When we're bored or lonely we fill the gap with many indulgences. And when we're stressed, we think of the problem as larger than ourselves. We lack the will to eat well or exercise because unhealthy habits give us a false sense of comfort. But while whiskey, cake or a cigarette may give us instant pleasure, when devoured mindlessly, they destroy us from within.

Eventually, our body tires of constant assaults and sends us messages—be it fatigue, pain or poor skin. But still we don't listen. Instead of changing habits, we look for instant solutions—a miracle serum, a chemical peel, antibiotics— anything to brighten up our stressed complexions. Great skincare and dermatological treatments will make our skin clearer. But none of it will last unless we learn to eat and live well. Even the act of drinking ten glasses of water will lead to clarity.

I'm not saying all indulgence is bad. Even an addiction to health is negative because it gives rise to fear. But we must indulge mindfully, with awareness. When we're not aware we tend to become gluttonous. And gluttony will always make us choose a burger over a home-cooked meal, and wine over water.

I too have struggled with my skin. I too have overindulged in things that were not good for me. Like the nine-step skincare routine, which made my delicate skin red and raw. Or the overpriced designer face oil that made my skin peel so badly that I had to use a steroid cream to halt the damage. I had to develop the habit of drinking water because these healthy habits didn't come naturally to me. If I had my way I'd laze around in bed all day with a cake in hand. Sugar is my guilty pleasure. So I'm familiar with the struggle and the anguish; cosmetics and treatments offer only topical relief.

Long-lasting transformation is possible only with food. Eating well takes care of not just physical but also our emotional health. Think of it like a daily medicine that heals us without side-effects. Once we eat with the intention of wellness and not just gratification, our skin will undergo a metamorphosis. From being beset with breakouts it will magically clear up, and that too for the long term.

In this part I've listed some medicinal herbs and common vegetables that help clarify the skin. They improve liver function and purify blood. However, some of these healers are extremely potent and must be taken in minuscule quantities. Choose one medicinal herb at a time. Because these ingredients are all about detoxification, it is essential to nourish the body with a wholesome diet first. Only then can we take these medicinal nutraceuticals. If we're starved, we're not ready for detoxification. This is why we must first energize and strengthen our body before we work to purify it.

12

NEEM

The most exciting time for me as a child was when my mother would open her trunk of saris. It had the softest silk chiffon *leheriya*s, rich, intricately woven Benarasis, the most delicate lace from Amritsar as well as blouses, trimmings, velvets and satin petticoats. Whenever we pulled a sari out of that precious trunk, a few dried neem leaves would flutter to the floor as my mother layered her precious silks and chiffons with fresh neem leaves to guard them against insects.

Neem is the magic bullet for health and beauty in India. We mix it into masks, drink it as tea and even use it to protect our clothes from infestation. It is because of this insecticidal quality that our revered neem is banned in Canada, and until recently wasn't authorized for use in the United Kingdom too. It is part poison after all. But all great healers have poisonous compounds and neem is no different. In fact, we love it for exactly the same reasons it is banned for.

Science

Scientists have now proved what Ayurveda always knew—
that neem has potent antifungal, antibacterial properties
along with being a strong insecticide. Modern science has also
found 140 compounds from the neem tree that can be used
for therapeutic purposes. These compounds (polysaccharides,
catechin, gallic acid and sodium nimbidate, among many
others) also work as anti-inflammatory agents. Because of
this, neem is used as a complementary treatment for diabetes
as it helps bring down blood sugar levels.

In 2012, Sonia Arora, an assistant professor at Kean
University, New Jersey, presented a paper at the experimental
biology conference in San Diego. According to her research,
neem attacks proteins that make new copies of the HIV virus.[1]
This powerful plant is currently being studied for its antiviral
properties to find a cure for HIV-AIDS. With such potential
to purify the body of bad microbes, neem should, at the very
least, be an essential component of every anti-acne routine.

Tradition

Neem is known as *sarva roga nivarini*—the cure for all
diseases. Each and every part of the tree is beneficial. Perhaps
that is the reason why the most potent concoctions have all
five parts of the tree—leaves, bark, root, fruit and flower.
It has been used for centuries in traditional medicine. The
leaves were eaten as a vegetable for inflammatory skin diseases
and in place of quinine to alleviate the symptoms of malaria.
When consumed it purifies the blood and provides relief from

skin diseases such as eczema and psoriasis. The paste of neem leaves and bark, when applied on a breakout, kills bacteria and fungus, thereby reducing the intensity of the pimple.

This ancient tree is revered for its cooling effect on the body. Because of this property, it has been used for problems caused by excess heat in the body that result in breakouts and blemishes. It increases immunity, removes toxins from the body and also boosts metabolism. A Sanskrit synonym for neem is *pichumard*—one that takes care of all skin disorders. Because it is antibacterial, it is great for oral hygiene too. Even today in villages neem twigs are used to keep the teeth healthy and free of decay. It is light, bitter, astringent and very cooling.

Neem is a pain reliever too. If you're tired, have leg cramps and muscle aches, you can massage the oil before you sleep to wake up refreshed in the morning. In addition, neem seed oil is very effective for premature greying and dandruff. Also, neem flowers can be used for any form of skin allergies. According to the *Charaka Samhita*, you can hand pound them and add to any face mask.

Application

Neem is extremely potent and must not be consumed for more than a month. When taken for a short period it can kill the bad bacteria. However, over the long term, it can kill the good bacteria in your gut and also have an anti-fertility effect.

If you have redness and urticaria (hives), pound 2–3 neem leaves with 1 crushed amla and 1 teaspoon of ghee and take it once a day after a meal. If you're suffering from hot flushes and feeling malaise and fever because of exhaustion, you can take any part of the neem tree and sprinkle it over lit coals to fumigate the room. The best way to do this would be using a *sambrani* burner.

Gut-Cleansing Neem Begun

4–5 neem leaves
1 small brinjal
Panchphoran (a pinch each of fenugreek, fennel, cumin, nigella and carom seeds)
1 teaspoon mustard oil
Salt to taste

- Heat the mustard oil till it smokes.
- Then add the panchphoran and cook till golden brown.
- Add the neem leaves, brinjal and salt and cook till the brinjal becomes soft and mushy.
- Consume this with the first morsel of food.
- This is a great antimicrobial agent for your gut.

Skin-Clearing Neem Steam

15–20 drops of cold pressed neem oil
A handful of crushed neem leaves (optional)

- Fill a steamer with water.
- Add the crushed neem leaves and neem oil to it.
- Then switch on the steamer and steam the face with it for 10-15 minutes. Follow with a cooling face pack.

- This is recommended for sensitive skin prone to acne, bumps and itchiness.

Purifying Neem Tea

2–3 neem leaves
½ an amla
1–2 peppercorns
½-inch piece ginger, crushed
1 teaspoon honey (optional)

- Crush the neem leaves with amla, peppercorns and crushed ginger.
- Boil this in 200 ml (a large glass) of water.
- After the water comes to a boil, take it off the heat and let the ingredients steep for 5 minutes.
- Strain and add honey, if required, for taste.
- In summer, avoid peppercorn because it is too hot.
- This works as a blood purifier—neem and ginger are detoxifiers and the other ingredients clear the channels for better absorption.

13

MANJISHTHA

Any Ayurvedic expert will talk ad nauseam about the skin-beautifying effects of manjishtha. A lot of people I met in the holistic field were so besotted with this herb that I finally caved in and ordered a jar of organic powder myself. I knew it cleared pigmentation, I knew it increased brightness and radiance, so when it was finally delivered, I scooped a hefty teaspoon of the powder into a bowl with a bit of Himalayan clay and aloe vera. So far so good. The mask was brick red and after washing it off, my face was too—red, and itchy.

It was only later that I found that only a pinch of this potent herb must be used at a time because it is very powerful. In fact, manjishtha works best as an extract or pre-prepared decoction—especially when consumed. This powerful herb is a blood purifier, antioxidant, depigmentor and an anti-inflammatory agent. Even though you may not have heard of it, it is a common addition in Ayurvedic face masks and creams. And in the world of Ayurveda, it is the ultimate beautifier.

Science

Also known as Indian madder, like other red fruits such as beetroot and pomegranate, manjishtha too is a powerful antioxidant and detoxifier. It not only helps purify the blood but also the lymphatic system. Its vast antioxidant capabilities help bring down inflammation, which helps calm and clear acne-prone skin. Research proves that manjishtha inhibits the growth of p.acnes bacteria, which is responsible for breakouts. In earlier times it was cultivated for the rich red pigments derived from its roots—the part that is actively used.

A smooth, acne-free complexion is just one of the innumerable benefits it offers. Manjishtha protects the cells, has radioprotective properties, helps reduce blood sugar—making it a great ally for diabetics—and also speeds up wound healing. Because of its high antioxidant content and diuretic properties, it also plays an important role in the management of hypertension and cardiovascular disease.

But what makes this herb really powerful is that it contains substantial amounts of anthraquinones (phenolic compounds that are present in its red-coloured roots). These stimulate digestion and also have an anti-tumour effect. It is because of these properties that manjishtha is now being studied as treatment for several diseases, including cancer.

Tradition

The great sage Charaka placed manjishtha in two categories—varnya (the herbs that improve the complexion) and *visaghna* (the detoxifiers). It is also a well-known rasayana or rejuvenator. When your skin is red, inflamed and burning, nothing clears it better than manjishtha—unless you use it wrongly like I did.

In Sanskrit it is also known as *tamravalli*—the climber with a copper hue. It has been mentioned that it is a brain-enhancing herb. This powerful ingredient works by detoxifying the blood and lymphatic system. It clears out any blockages in circulation so that toxins do not build up and cleans the liver. Because it works like a mild laxative, it cleans the colon too. It works especially well during summer when your skin and eyes have the tendency to burn.

Manjishtha's primary tastes are bitter, astringent and sweet. The bitter taste works directly on detoxifying the liver, while the astringent taste helps cool the blood. Sweet is the most nourishing and cooling taste. So this herb powerfully detoxifies, cools, unclogs circulatory channels and nourishes the cells and tissues.

Application

The roots of this plant have been traditionally used to heal various skin conditions such as eczema, psoriasis, acne and even burns. Its external clarifying effects are boosted when taken internally as a supplement or decoction. As mentioned earlier, the best way to use this herb is in a pre-prepared extract, in combination with other herbs. Therefore, manjishtha is usually found along with other herbs in supplements. Just look for it in the ingredient list. Any Ayurvedic medicine or supplement that claims to improve skin will contain manjishtha.

The root is an excellent pitta pacifier (excess pitta shows up as red, inflamed skin). It takes away all the pitta abnormalities—breakouts, acne and rosacea—and makes your skin glow. It is warming in nature, so it also pacifies kapha that manifests as excess weight.

People with acne or old scars can add it to face packs, or use *maha manjishtha kwath* (a liquid medicinal syrup made in combination with other herbs such as neem and turmeric) to make tea. Take 25 g of the *kwath* and add four times water and boil. Once it is ¼th of the original volume, drink it with a little bit of *mishri* to make it palatable.

Note: People who suffer from diarrhoea should not consume it because it increases bowel movement.

Tone-Clearing Manjishtha Lep

A pinch of manjishtha
1 teaspoon red sandalwood powder
½ teaspoon washed red lentils (*masoor* dal)
½ teaspoon fig tree bark powder (optional)
½ teaspoon *lodhra* powder (optional)
A splash of rose water
½ teaspoon or more of aloe vera gel to make a paste

- Mix the manjishtha and red sandalwood powder.
- Soak the red lentils and when soft make a paste. Add ½ teaspoon of this paste into the powder.
- If you have fig tree bark powder and lodhra powder, add these into it.
- Add the rose water and aloe vera gel to turn it into a paste.
- Apply on the face and leave it on till it starts drying. Then rub it off.
- This helps detoxify and even out the skin tone. It is adopted from a *varnya lep* in *Ashtanga Hridayam*. Most of these ingredients are varnya (skin-boosting) themselves.

14

KATUKI

Whenever there is a skin problem there is a high chance that it is connected to the liver. Our liver filters the blood, removes chemicals and metabolizes drugs and hormones in the body. It also synthesizes protein and produces bile that helps in digestion. When the liver is sluggish, you won't be able to digest food and may suffer from constipation. A poorly functioning liver cannot synthesize drugs or hormones properly. Therefore there may be signs of hormonal imbalance such as mood swings, breakouts or menstrual problems. When the body is full of toxins, hormonally imbalanced or when our digestive system isn't functioning properly, it leads to poor skin, eczema, breakouts and rashes.

But there's good news too. Your liver is one organ that can regenerate itself. So if you choose to take care of it and nourish it well, unless severely damaged, it will reward you by becoming healthy again.

Katuki (*kutki* or *katuka*) is the most powerful liver tonic. Like turmeric, it is also a rhizome, but it grows high in the

Himalayas. It can detoxify the liver before or after taking toxins (e.g. painkillers or alcohol) and also helps treat long-standing conditions such as fatty liver and hepatitis C.

Katuki literally means bitter, so like everything else that enhances liver function, this too is immensely unpalatable. Still, I would strongly recommend that you put aside flavour because it is the ultimate tool to improve all internal functions and thereby clarify your complexion.

Science

The efficacy of this rhizome can be credited to compounds called kutkin. While scientists haven't been able to figure out exactly how they work, they're still credited with anti-inflammatory, immunity-modulating properties. This means that katuki will not just reduce irritations but also prevent allergies. Perhaps this is the reason why it's such a handy tool to fight skin conditions such as acne and psoriasis.

In a study published way back in 1989, it was shown that 27 per cent of subjects who suffered from vitiligo found that taking katuki extract completely resolved their symptoms.[1]

The root contains powerful antioxidants that help improve cardiovascular conditions and other lifestyle diseases. It helps lower cholesterol, unclogs the arteries and its anti-inflammatory action aids in treating arthritis.

Tradition

The great sage Charaka placed this powerful herb in the category of *bhedniya mahakashaya*—herbs that can purge the liver and cleanse the colon. Bitter is the coldest and the most detoxifying taste in Ayurveda, so katuki has an immensely cooling effect on the body. It also falls under the category of *lekhaniya*—herbs that have a scraping effect on the insides and cause weight loss. It is extremely light to digest, improves metabolism and is useful in cases of diabetes (it seems all bitter herbs are).

Even in Ayurveda it is useful in allergies and asthma. You can think of katuki as a herbal antibiotic. In earlier times it was used to bring down high fever. It helps balance the digestive system, helping equally in cases of acute diarrhoea and constipation. Because it cools down the body, prevents allergies, detoxifies the liver, scrapes the insides for toxic waste and balances digestion, it is extremely effective in clarifying the complexion.

Application

Only a pinch of katuki should be consumed daily. Both science and tradition prove its liver detoxifying and fortifying properties. Therefore, when taken in the right manner, it will improve every function of your body. Take one pinch along with any juice or water. You can also take a pinch each of katuki and liquorice (*yashti madhu*) with a little bit of mishri. This combination is safe for anyone to consume and helps improve circulation and alleviates liver and kidney issues.

15

TRIPHALA

Can a digestive make you sleep better?

I'd heard about the colon-cleansing, antioxidant powers of this tri-herb Ayurvedic concoction (made with amla, *haritaki* and *bhibhitaki*), but sleep was an unexpected benefit. By sleep I mean a deep, uninterrupted, dreamless 7 hours. I eat a teaspoon just before sleeping and chug it down with water. I may read for 10 minutes or so, but after that my lids get heavy. Sleep comes swiftly, without any twisting and turning. It has become my nightly ritual for completely different reasons.

My grandfather used to make triphala at home. He would get all the three herbs—amla, haritaki and bhibhitaki—and grind them together in equal portions. If there was anyone who was the idol for health and wellness it was him. He used to call it the ultimate healer, saying that if anyone had a spoonful of triphala every day, they would live a long and healthy life. Well, at least he proved this theory with his own example.

It has been proved over and over again that the health of your colon is directly linked to the glow on your face. Poor elimination leads to acidity, bloating, flatulence, breakouts and sensitivities. If your colon is clean and healthy, elimination is smoother. When that happens you get a flat belly, clear skin and sparkling eyes. But I digress. The amazing benefit of triphala is that not only does it clear your digestive tract, it also cleans you especially well on the days when you've gone on an unhealthy binge.

Science

For starters, it is packed with vitamin C courtesy the amla, which also contains iron and B vitamins, among other precious nutrients. Haritaki, the second ingredient, is the best digestive herb and the ultimate detoxifier. The last herb in this trio is bhibhitaki. It is also packed with vitamin C and minerals such as selenium and iron. It fights infections, clears the respiratory system and relives inflammation. A combination of the three is a time-tested recipe that works on both prevention and cure. Both animal and human studies have shown that triphala can help reduce body fat[1] and weight[2] and control cholesterol[3] and glucose levels,[4] thereby boosting immunity.

This amazing churna is packed with antioxidants, including capillary-strengthening flavonoids. It protects the liver and has antiviral, antibacterial, anti-allergic and anti-carcinogenic properties. It improves circulation, lowers blood pressure and also shows wound-healing capacity. When taken regularly year after year, you will see improvement in health and immunity.

Tradition

In Ayurveda, triphala is known as a rasayana (anti-ageing rejuvenator). It balances all the three doshas and is therefore safe for everyone. You can take it throughout your life to improve skin, hair and overall health. Its functions include improving digestion, scraping the insides for old accumulations, absorbing fluids from the intestines, working against haemorrhoids and improving the absorption of other herbs. In addition, it also improves the downward flow of air (or vata) which is responsible for elimination.

This churna contains all six Ayurvedic tastes—sweet, astringent, sour, salty, pungent and bitter. So depending on what you've eaten during the day, one of these tastes would be more dominant when you eat it at night. At this point I must say that triphala is just the most difficult nutraceutical that you're ever going to stomach. Not that it tastes like feet or anything (trust me, there are foods like that), but just bitter, sour and dry as hell, especially in the beginning. Over time I've learnt to enjoy its taste. From bitter and pungent, I now taste more of its astringency. So the point is, when you binge it will taste more bitter than usual, almost like a little rap on the knuckles for being unhealthy. And if you have eaten healthy all day, then it will be less bitter and more sour, with a sweet aftertaste. Interesting, isn't it?

Western medicine looks at every element or each ingredient on its own. But Ayurveda looks at everything in combination.

It's an art to really know what goes well together—to know the combinations that boost a herb's potency. Amla with its high vitamin C is an immunity booster, haritaki is a mild laxative and bhibhitaki takes out any obstruction in the channels of your body. When the three are combined, together they give a boost of antioxidants, work as colon cleansers, nourish the tissues and organs, add luminosity to the skin and strength to the hair, purify the blood, help in weight loss and improve bone health, among many other benefits.

Application

These days I make a tea with ½ a teaspoon of triphala mixed in hot water every night. After I mix the powder I let it sit for 10–15 minutes or even longer. This should be the last thing you drink before bed, a couple of hours after dinner. This is the traditional way of drinking this powerful superfood, and this also makes its properties even more potent. Good luck sipping on this hot, bitter tea. But if you can stomach it, then this is the most wonderful way to drink it. It's similar to a basic supplement like calcium or fish oil which, over time, really strengthens, nourishes and detoxifies the body. And it really helps you 'go' in the mornings. But the great part about this churna, as is the case with any Ayurvedic herb, is that there are so many ways to take it, each with its own unique set of benefits.

To use this wonderful churna as a rejuvenator, take 1–2 teaspoons of it with milk. When taken with milk or ghee (in the same quantity as the triphala) it improves strength, vitality and immunity. You can take this concoction early in the morning to kick-start your day. You can also take a teaspoon with warm water at least one and a half hours after dinner. This way it will work as a mild laxative. If you want to improve your appetite, take it with warm water an hour before your meal. If you want to improve IBS (irritable bowel syndrome), you can take a spoonful in the morning with a pinch of rock salt. If you have a cough, just add 3–4 fresh tulsi leaves to a teaspoon of the powder. Keep the mixture in your mouth and chew it so that the juices run down your throat to soothe it. In fact, triphala can also be used to gargle at the first signs of a sore throat. And you can eat it with jaggery to detoxify the body.

Coming back to sleep, empirical evidence suggests that too much of this blend can cause insomnia. However, there are many people (like me) who report better sleep with a spoonful before bed. A spoonful is not excessive. Do keep in mind that you must not use triphala if you're fasting, have gastric ulcers, heart burn, excessive weight loss or very dry skin. If you have loose stools when you take it on an empty stomach, then take it after a meal.

Make your own triphala

Firstly, the three ingredients—haritaki, bhibhitaki and amla—should be free of moisture or dirt. Dry them in the sun for a day to ensure that they are fully dry. Then powder the ingredients in a spice blender in the ratio 1:2:4 for a higher ratio of antioxidants.

16

TURMERIC (HALDI)

First turmeric was considered good, then there was news that curcumin (the main active ingredient) wasn't that good at all and now there's talk that it is wonderful again. I don't understand the concept of separating a molecule or a single nutrient from a plant and selling it as a supplement. Even if curcumin is the active ingredient in turmeric, there are many other elements that together give this rhizome its superpowers. Did you know that 100 kg of turmeric produces 3–3.5 kg of 95 per cent curcumin? What about the other antioxidants, flavonoids, vitamins and minerals in it?

Science

We Indians have been using this spice in our curries since time immemorial. However, most of the research has been conducted on curcumin, a powerful polyphenol that decreases the risk of cancer, works as an antioxidant, anti-inflammatory agent and also reduces blood fat and sugar levels. However, turmeric is more than just curcumin. It also contains many other phytochemicals including demethoxycurcumin (helps in hypertension, along with lung, breast and ovarian cancers), tumerones (help in reducing inflammation, serum lipid levels, gastric ulcers, diabetes) and tumenorols (anti-inflammatory, antioxidant compounds). Turmeric also contains minerals such as manganese, iron, copper and potassium that make it worth more than just its curcumin content.

Tradition

Turmeric, haldi or *haridra* is also called *nisha*—beautiful as a moonlit night. Other synonyms for it are *kanchani* (that which shines like dazzling gold) and *yoshit priya* (that which is loved by women). In olden days shopkeepers would keep mounds of bright yellow turmeric outside their stores to attract customers. Therefore it's also called *haat vilasini*— that which makes the shop attractive. Needless to say, it is one of the most effective antimicrobial, antibacterial detoxifiers that enhances the complexion as well. It is warming, so it should not be applied directly on the face and definitely not on sensitive skin. You need to use turmeric in a cooling base like *multani mitti* (fuller's earth); otherwise it will aggravate acne.

Of course it is healing and antiseptic but few know that it is a pain reliever too. It's no wonder that many sportspeople drink turmeric milk regularly to soothe injuries and get relief from aches and pains.

In Ayurveda, turmeric is said to improve the skin quality and impart a golden hue to the complexion. It provides relief from itchiness, worm or microbe infection and has a scraping quality that detoxifies the internal organs. While it is light and dry in terms of digestion, it is hot in potency. Therefore, unless a herbalist or doctor advises, you must avoid supplementing this spice in summer. It is perfectly fine to use it in food. In fact turmeric is said to reduce carcinogens when applied to meat before grilling it.

Application

The best way to consume any food product is in its whole form and in the traditional manner. It has been found that when turmeric is taken with pepper, it increases the bioavailability of curcumin manifold. Even taking it with fat increases the absorption. This is why we add it in our curries and drink it in milk—the fat in milk and the oil and spices in curries help the body sop up its healing abilities.

I find that taking turmeric (not curcumin) supplements has really boosted my immunity. The one that I use has *trikatu* (an Ayurvedic churna made of black pepper, long pepper and dried ginger). I take it with food and fish oil capsules to add the fat element. It has kept me away from the common cold and flu all winter. I also take turmeric mixed with ghee and pepper to heal yoga injuries because it is best for unseen, internal bruises that can only be felt.

There are so many varieties of the turmeric plant. I heard from someone that the turmeric from Meghalaya (*lakadong* turmeric) is the most potent because it has high levels of curcumin. I asked a friend to get me some, and when I saw it I realized that there could be some truth in that claim because that variety had the brightest, almost orange, yellow colour.

But then there's also the really gentle white variety and *kasturi manjal* (the wild form of haldi) that has been used for years in traditional skincare.

Turmeric should be used in limited quantities in face masks. I find that when I apply too much it stains my skin and makes it prone to rashes and breakouts. I think it is too much of a good thing and must be used only as a small component in a recipe. For instance, you can mix aloe vera and honey and add a pinch of turmeric. This is a highly potent ingredient, whether you eat or apply it. I remember one friend who took 1 whole teaspoon of turmeric on an empty stomach. Within half an hour she was feeling hot and uncomfortable, and later that day she broke out into a few spots. So use it wisely.

However, if turmeric is part of your diet, you don't need to supplement it if you're healthy. I was taking it to heal from a surgery for endometriosis. Even though I felt like I'd healed from the outside, I still felt raw and tender, and nothing is better to heal internal injuries than this wonderful Indian spice.

Immunity-Boosting Turmeric Milk

1 inch fresh turmeric root, crushed
1 cup milk (nut or dairy)
¼ teaspoon black peppercorn, crushed

- Boil the milk with the turmeric root and black peppercorn.
- Bring to a boil. Simmer for a couple of minutes to really extract the flavour.
- Strain and drink. You can even use nut milk with this recipe if you are allergic to lactose.

Other Varieties

White Turmeric

Amba haldi, *zedoary* or white turmeric has seen a recent surge in popularity because it is part of some green, organic skincare products. It contains the maximum amount of essential oils and hence is the most aromatic variant of turmeric. It has a camphor- or mango-like fragrance because of which it is very popular for use in pickles and jams. It is especially good for irritated, itching skin and doesn't stain the skin as much as yellow turmeric. It contains the same antimicrobial, anti-inflammatory and blood-purifying properties; however, it is less reactive. It also stimulates digestion, works as a diuretic, improves respiratory disorders and regulates body temperature too. When applied on the skin, it has a cooling and healing effect and therefore makes a great addition to face masks.

White Turmeric Brightening Mask

1 tablespoon white turmeric powder
1 tablespoon rose powder
1 tablespoon kaolin clay powder
Enough rose water to make a paste
½ teaspoon honey (optional)

- Mix the white turmeric with rose and kaolin clay powders.
- Add a bit of rose water to make a paste and apply over the face and neck till the decolletage.

- You can enhance the mask by adding several drops of a good quality essential oil like supercritically extracted sea buckthorn oil.
- You can also add a touch of honey for its moisturizing and antibacterial properties.
- Wash it just when it begins to dry.
- White turmeric is anti-inflammatory, but has the added benefit of brightening the skin. Rose powder helps combat rosacea and balances the skin tone.

Wild Turmeric

Kasturi manjal or wild turmeric is a popular ingredient in traditional Indian skincare. Its antibacterial and anti-inflammatory properties help fight acne, while its antioxidant composition helps reduce wrinkles and sun damage. It balances excessive oil production on the face and reduces burning and itching on the skin, especially due to insect bites. It is not used for internal consumption, however, its gentle composition makes it a popular addition to children's ubtans. It doesn't stain your skin as much and that's why it is used so much in external preparations. It also helps in cases of urticaria (hives), making this variation of turmeric one of the most prized traditional ingredients in skincare.

Kasturi Manjal Glow Mask

¼ teaspoon kasturi manjal
¼ teaspoon freshly ground neem leaves
¼ teaspoon sandalwood powder

1–2 saffron strands
Enough milk to make a paste
A splash of rosewater (optional)

- Mix the kasturi manjal, freshly ground neem leaves, sandalwood powder and saffron with milk.
- Make a paste. You can also add a little rosewater.
- Apply on the face and wash before it is completely dry.
- This helps add glow, targets bad bacteria and evens out the skin tone.

17

GINGER AND GARLIC

These two ingredients that form the basis of Indian cooking are also the two most powerful anti-inflammatory, antioxidant agents. I have always believed that traditional food combinations aren't just for taste. They always have some rationale behind them. Take, for instance, ginger–garlic paste, which forms the base for the masala in most Indian curries.

Interestingly, while both spices are warming in nature, ginger is purely sattvic, whereas garlic is rajasic and tamasic. Let me simplify this for you: sattva, rajas and tamas are the three gunas or qualities that govern all life. Sattvic foods calm and centre the mind. They are preferred by yogis who need to be detached from materialistic attractions to stay on the spiritual path. Rajasic foods, on the other hand, are energizing. Unlike sattvic foods, they give you the motivation or energy to achieve more from the outside world. Because of this they work for ambitious people. Tamas means laziness, darkness or inertia. But we require tamasic energies too. After all it's only when we are tamasic or lazy that we can go to sleep.

While we all strive to be more sattvic, rajas and tamas are also essential for maintaining the equilibrium. Because of this reason the combination of ginger–garlic paste is extremely balanced and, needless to say, highly nutritious. Even separately these pungent foods are healing and clarifying, especially when used specifically to cure a condition. Ginger is my mother's favourite spice—she adds a handful of it in lentils, soups and even saag. Garlic is my personal favourite—I burn it for smokiness, roast to make it sweet and gooey or chop it finely to toss into salads for that extra bite.

Strong flavours in natural ingredients are a sign of their potency. In Ayurveda, the taste of an ingredient is an indicator of its therapeutic capability, and each of the six tastes (sweet, sour, salty, bitter, pungent, astringent) has a different purpose. Think about it: don't you find eating desserts comforting? That's because sweet taste is the most soothing and nourishing. Or when you eat something astringent (like raw fruit), doesn't it feel clarifying after a fatty meal? Pungent tastes like that of ginger and garlic stimulate digestion, absorption and elimination, boost metabolism, purify the blood and detoxify the body. It's no wonder then that eating ginger and garlic is beneficial for both skin and hair.

Ginger

If you go to any spa, ginger, lemon and honey tea will definitely be on the menu. There will be a lot of ginger in your food and in your green juice. It will also be pickled as an accompaniment. The reason for this is that ginger is highly effective in bringing down inflammation. It also helps clear the internal channels and delivers the benefit of any preparation right to the tissues. The best part is that ginger is commonly available and so easy to use. I feel that when we eat without appreciation, the effects of food get slightly diminished. So the next time you drink a cup of strong ginger tea, remind yourself of all its healing benefits and you'll find that it nourishes you better.

Science

Ginger holds a vast antioxidant profile (surpassed only by pomegranate and certain types of berries). It has vitamin C, polyphenols, beta-carotene and flavonoids, all working together to make this a food that fights damage. The active ingredients in ginger are phenolic compounds called gingerols. They are so effective in bringing down inflammation and swelling that this spice is strongly recommended to reduce symptoms of arthritis. A 2017 study published in the journal *Cancer Management and Research* shows that 6-gingerol helps protect the body against free radicals and also increases antioxidant activity in the body.[1] At the end of the day our skin is just a reflection of our internal health. Inflammation is the main cause behind most diseases and poor skin condition. Think about it—acne, psoriasis and eczema are all inflammatory in nature. By eating and cooking with ginger we can help the body heal itself.

Tradition

In Ayurveda, ginger is known as *vishwabhesaj* or universal medicine. Its exalted place in the traditional kitchen is well deserved because it builds up digestive fire and gets rid of ama or un-metabolized food that circulates as toxins in the body. The accumulation of this waste is the main cause of disease according to Ayurveda.

Ginger is a purely sattvic food, which brings about the qualities of balance and calm. Because it is a warming spice, it increases circulation, promotes sweating, removes phlegm from the lungs and aids in easy breathing. This spice also enhances the effect of any other herb that it is combined with. So if you combine ginger with neem, it will reach the blood to purify it. If you combine it with, say, pepper, it will help clear the digestive tract.

It has a hot potency so it cuts down toxins, but it has a sweet post-digestive effect (called vipaka in Ayurveda) because of which it soothes and nourishes the tissues. Ginger on its own or combined with other food helps in detoxification and better absorption of nutrients. It is used extensively not just in India but also in many other cultures around the world.

Application

The warming effects of ginger are well known. Whenever you have a cold, a cup of ginger tea instantly makes you feel better. My friend, who regularly practises yoga, rubs plain ginger juice directly on sprains. The heating effect of this medicinal root goes deep into the tissues, while its anti-inflammatory qualities help soothe redness and swelling.

Dried ginger powder (sonth) is also used in cases of gastrointestinal distress. If you feel gassy and bloated, try rubbing the powder on your stomach. It is folk knowledge, something that my grandmother recommends, but it is the best remedy for digestive distress. While fresh ginger is heating and ideal for winter months, dry ginger is comparatively more cooling and therefore more suited for summer.

I love ginger because it is easily available and even more easy to use. You can add it to food, make a tea, pickle it or eat it like a candy. Pickling and fermenting ginger is an excellent idea. Because it is packed with fibre, it works as a wonderful prebiotic, or food for the good bacteria in your gut. Fermentation also makes it a natural probiotic, which just doubles the benefits.

Garlic

I read online that rubbing a slice of garlic directly on a breakout helps flatten it and prevents it from coming back. I would never, ever rub anything quite so pungent (neither ginger nor garlic) directly on my face. It could increase redness and cause my sensitive skin to burn. But taken internally, garlic is extremely fortifying for the body. It also works as an extremely powerful antioxidant, which means it helps bring down irritation and redness.

Science

The main component of garlic is allicin, which is responsible for its distinct smell and flavour. This compound decomposes as soon as it comes in touch with a free radical (in the air) to produce potent antioxidants. In one study a scientist said that they had not seen any other compound, either natural or synthetic, react so quickly as an antioxidant.[2]

Garlic is used by people suffering from cardiovascular disease and even cancer. It contains compounds not found in many foods that help detoxify the body at a cellular level and nourish the joints and connective tissue. Anything that contains sulphur is beneficial for skin conditions such as acne. Besides sulphur, garlic also contains manganese, vitamins C and B6, along with trace minerals such as copper and selenium that are essential for healthy skin. A great benefit of garlic is that it reduces toxin-related damage and also helps support our internal detoxification system.

Tradition

Purely sattvic diets in India are always free of garlic and onion. A colleague once told me that he got rid of anger within six months of removing these two pungent additions from his diet. But that said, I feel that garlic must only be avoided if you are on the path to becoming a sage or really want to manage your anger. Because in all other aspects, garlic's benefits outweigh its 'risks'. It is considered a rajasic or energizing food. There are no problems with such foods. In *Ayurveda of the Mind*, author Dr David Frawley writes that to get out of a depressive low energy or tamasic (lazy) state, one must first energize the body with rajasic elements. So garlic is beneficial in many ways.

It contains all five tastes except sour, meaning it nourishes and detoxifies the body and boosts immunity and metabolism. In Ayurveda, garlic is also known as *kushtaghna* (that which is useful for skin conditions) and *jantujit* (that which gets rid of microbes). It also cuts down ama and clears the internal channels so that whatever goes in next can be absorbed properly. This is why a simple dal and rice meal is so nutritious—it contains ginger or garlic that cleanses the body before nourishing it with proteins, carbohydrates and amino acids. Simple, yet genius. Now that's something to appreciate the next time you sit down for an Indian meal.

Application

A lot of people eat a clove of garlic on an empty stomach in the morning to reduce the risk of cardiovascular disease and improve complexion. There's nothing wrong with it, but it would be better if it is first lightly crushed and then left in the open for 10–15 minutes. During this time the oxygen in the air helps the enzyme alliinase convert alliin into allicin, which is the active ingredient responsible for garlic's superpowers. Even when using it in curries or pasta, chop or crush garlic, then leave it out in the open for 10–15 minutes before you cook with it.

If you have hyperacidity, eating a raw garlic clove on an empty stomach will make your condition worse. But you can still get the benefits by cooking 1–2 cloves of garlic in a cup each of water and milk. When the water evaporates and only the milk remains wait till it becomes lukewarm to drink this infusion. You must keep in mind that garlic cloves should be consumed on an empty stomach only during winter.

18

ALOE VERA

There's everything to love about this succulent. Aloe vera has saved my skin on multiple occasions. It has healed cuts, severe burns and even mild acne. I apply aloe vera as a night cream on days when my skin looks red, inflamed and bumpy. It looks clear the morning after, and by evening, even the tiny bumps dry up completely. I keep several aloe plants in my house. I find that it works well to just slap the pulp on my face when no other skincare works. It can also be added to face masks for a cooling and hydrating effect. Personally, I like to apply aloe vera rather than eat it. I feel that the results are far better when applied and also much quicker. There are so many wonderful herbs that can be eaten, but only very few that are effective when applied straight up, like aloe vera.

Science

One look at the nutritional profile of aloe vera and you know why it's such a panacea for skin problems. It contains vitamins A, C, E and B12, twenty of the twenty-two amino acids required by humans and also skin-friendly minerals such as copper, selenium and zinc, among many others. It also has eight enzymes that break down sugar and fat (one of them also brings down inflammation on the skin), salicylic acid (to reduce breakouts) and saponins (cleansing, antiseptic agents).

Research has proved that aloe gel is effective on first- and second-degree burns and also speeds up wound healing. Lovneet told me about an incident that she witnessed when she was studying in naturopathy school. Someone with terrible burns had been hospitalized and the doctors used water, aloe vera and clay to heal her burns. First they applied chilled, damp bandages for 15 minutes. Then they put on a thick layer of clay that was kept on for another 15–20 minutes. So terrible were her burns that when the chilled bandages and cold clay were removed both were steaming because they pulled out the excessive heat. The last step was to apply a thick layer of aloe vera to really heal the skin. In about ten days her burns were almost cured. That is the power of nature.

Preliminary studies show that the gel may be effective in reducing the symptoms of psoriasis. The application of aloe also helps in seborrhoeic dermatitis and acne. One Korean study found that ingesting aloe vera gel improved the elasticity of the skin and reduced wrinkles too.[1] Studies also show that the glucomann (a polysaccharide) and gibberellin (a growth hormone) in aloe vera increase collagen synthesis when eaten or applied.[2]

Tradition

The Ayurvedic name for aloe vera is *kumari* or young girl. The name probably comes from its miraculous anti-ageing properties, and also because the plant looks plump and succulent even when it's old. It also helps in amenorrhoea— the absence of (or missed) periods. Aloe is also called *ghiritkumari* because its texture is as soft as ghee. Its primary taste is bitter, which is the most cooling and detoxifying taste. Aloe is considered a rasayana (anti-ageing elixir) and is used to treat everything from tumours to acne, boils, burns, wounds, ulcers and fibroids. It balances all the three doshas, improves immunity, reduces hair fall and dandruff and enhances tissue regeneration, which is why it is so effective for skin problems. Traditionally it was also used to reduce blood sugar, boost immunity and purify the body by aiding liver function.

Application

The best part about aloe vera is that it's so versatile. It hydrates dry skin, heals pimples, reduces redness, soothes burns and makes the skin glow. It can be eaten, or applied like a cream or a mask on the face or hair. My only apprehension in eating it is that people sometimes overdo the quantity. If you eat more than the required dosage or if the quality is bad, it can cause abdominal discomfort. Instead of eating bottled or packaged aloe vera just mix 1–2 teaspoons of the gel in water and drink it on an empty stomach. While eating or applying, take care to remove the yellow goop and keep only the transparent clear gel.

::

Did you know that aloe vera makes a great vaginal wash?

Just mix 2 teaspoons of aloe vera juice (taken from fresh pulp) in warm water along with a pinch of rock salt and use it as a wash. This is excellent for people who suffer from recurrent infections.

::

Traditionally, a lot of people eat aloe stir-fried with salt and turmeric as a subzi. While this is fine for most people, especially women who have delayed periods, it should not be eaten by women who bleed excessively during menstruation. Aloe is heavy, slimy, sticky and heating, so consuming it may make heavy periods worse. Interestingly, it is cooling when applied, which is why I prefer to use it for application alone.

While aloe is soothing and calming on most skin types, there is a small percentage of people who are allergic to it. Therefore, it's always prudent to do a patch test before applying it directly.

Super-Shine Aloe Hair Mask

2 fresh red hibiscus flowers
4 hibiscus leaves
¼ cup fresh aloe vera pulp
1 tablespoon liquorice (*mulethi* or *yashti madhu*)

1 tablespoon dried amla powder
2–3 tablespoons honey (optional)

- Make a paste of the hibiscus flowers, leaves and aloe vera pulp.
- Add the liquorice and dried amla powders to it.
- You can add honey too if you have very dry hair.
- Just apply it on the hair and scalp. Do not massage. This will give nourishment to the scalp and to the keratin in the strands.

Aloe Clearing Skin Lep

1 tablespoon aloe vera gel (scooped out of the leaf)
1 tablespoon multani mitti
A pinch of turmeric power or fresh turmeric paste
1 teaspoon honey
A few drops of rosewater

- Make a paste with the aloe vera gel, multani mitti powder, turmeric powder, honey and rosewater.
- Apply it evenly on the face and neck for 15 minutes.
- Wash with water and pat dry.
- It is suitable for all skin types and can be used once a week.
- This lep is an excellent remedy to soothe tired and problem skin.

19

TURNIPS AND RADISHES

One of the great joys of winter is the amazing array of in-season root vegetables. Everyone loves carrots and beets because they're such amazing beauty foods. Carrots are packed with beta carotene, which is a precursor to vitamin A that is essential for great skin. I also know for a fact that one of India's best wellness centres serves beetroot juice to be taken on an empty stomach because it detoxifies the intestines. But poor turnips and radishes are often ignored and that's probably because of their taste. Turnips especially can be really bland when cooked. So in a world where everything from make-up to flavours work in the extreme, not many appreciate its delicate, simple taste. Radishes, on the other hand, can be a bit too sharp. Even I took many years to warm up to these extremely beneficial root vegetables. In my house turnips and radishes are enjoyed all winter. My grandfather believed that turnips especially had the power to boost health and longevity.

I became interested in turnips and radishes after my friend who also has endometriosis told me about their immensely detoxifying properties. She drinks radish juice quite regularly because she believes that it removes the excess oestrogen (that could worsen endometriosis symptoms) from her liver. This is just her own conclusion based on her research. Still, the reason these two veggies clarify the skin is because they detoxify the liver.

Like other root vegetables, turnips and radishes also contain a lot of fibre. Fibrous foods are the best cleansing agents, serve as food for good bacteria and also clean out the colon. If your GI tract is not clean, it's very difficult to have clear skin.

Radishes

Radishes are the ultimate beauty food. They're extremely low in calories. In fact, they're a negative calorie food. This means you're burning fat while eating them. They also contain vitamin C which increases collagen production, tonnes of fibre and several other minerals including magnesium and manganese.

Science

The main components of radish are isothiocyanates, which are sulphur-based chemical compounds found in all cruciferous vegetables such as cabbage, cauliflower, broccoli and kale. These isothiocyanates neutralize carcinogens that helps in lowering the risk of certain cancers.

Studies have shown that enzymes in radishes help protect the liver.[1] Because they contain coenzyme Q10, they also help prevent type 2 diabetes.[2] CoQ10 is a natural antioxidant which is found in every cell of our bodies. It helps generate cellular energy, fights against oxidative stress and prevents tissue damage. Low levels of this compound have been linked to diabetes, heart disease and certain types of cancers. Both the vegetable and leaves contain this antioxidant. Because CoQ10 is fat-soluble, it also makes sense to stir-fry the greens and roots with a little bit of oil and eat it as a side.

Radishes help in the production and flow of bile, enzymes and acids that aid digestion. This is perhaps the reason they are suggested as an alternative treatment for jaundice because they help the liver perform its functions well. We know that a healthy liver and effective digestion are the basis of clear skin. In addition, radishes also have a protein that has antifungal properties. Known as RsAFP2, it helps destroy the colonies of candida fungus that cause poor digestion, migraines and inflamed, irritated skin.

Tradition

Radish is an energizing, warming food that has been traditionally used to treat gastrointestinal disorders. Its primary tastes are pungent and bitter. Pungent flavours rekindle the digestive fire, give clarity to the senses, reduce inflammation and allergies, fight germs, increase blood circulation, purify the blood and improve the skin. Bitter taste, as we already know, is hugely detoxifying. Both these flavours help clear stagnant wastes (ama) in the body and cleanse the blood.

In Ayurveda the small radish is considered light and easy to digest while the large radish is heavy. Therefore, the small radish is best eaten raw, while the large radish when cooked with oil helps balance all the three doshas.

Application

Radishes can be stir-fried with their leaves in mustard oil and salt. If you don't like them raw, try cooking them with greens—it makes them taste quite delicious. In fact cooking with a bit of fat helps the absorption of oil-soluble vitamins A, E and K. Use only young radishes for juicing.

Skin Detox Elixir

- One really good cleansing juice combination is radish juice with fennel, orange, celery and cucumber.
- Use all in equal parts.
- These vegetables may not be as sweet as beetroots or carrots, but if you want clear skin they must be a part of your diet.

Radish Stir Fry

1 large cup of radish, chopped with leaves
½ teaspoon carom seeds (ajwain)
2–3 tablespoons mustard oil

- Separate the radish leaves and roots.
- Heat the mustard oil. When it smokes, add the ajwain seeds.
- When the seeds splutter, add the radish. Stir-fry for a few minutes. I like to keep them crunchy so I don't cook

them all the way through. Right at the end add the greens and stir-fry for 10–15 seconds. Take them off the heat.

Turnips

Being from the same family, turnips also have a similar nutritional profile. They're packed with vitamin C, beta-carotene and B vitamins, along with several phytonutrients that help protect you from environmental toxins. They also have high amounts of sulphur-based compounds that work against acne.

Science

Turnip greens are hugely nutritious. They're in the top ten vitamin A–rich foods, and also contain vitamins K, C, E and B6, along with minerals such as copper, manganese and fibre. However, care must be taken not to overcook them. They're rich in dietary nitrates, which are basically compounds that are found in most vegetables. By themselves nitrates have no effect but when absorbed by the body they are converted into nitrites that are known to relax blood vessels. A 2016 study published in the *British Journal of Clinical Pharmacology* actually found that vegetables rich in nitrates help lower blood pressure, among many other vascular benefits.[3]

Turnips are also extremely high in fibre and low in fat. Because of this reason they help improve digestion and keep the colon clear. However, they have lesser insoluble fibre as compared to radishes so they won't cause bloating or burning. When cooked they're easier on the colon.

Tradition

The primary tastes of turnip are pungent and astringent, which means that along with the effects of the former they help decongest the body, scrape away internal impurities, heal wounds and cleanse the mucous membranes with the astringent taste. Even in traditional medicine, turnips are considered cleansing for the liver, gall bladder, lymph and blood. There's no doubt that with their cleansing and detoxifying properties, this vegetable will help clarify and improve your complexion.

Application

I make a watery turnip curry to eat with rice. It's really bland but I love it for its incredible lightness. On days when I eat dinner late it's the ideal meal. You can add young turnips into a salad and add cubes of mature turnips into soups. They are also great substitutes for potatoes in a traditional mash recipe as they have lesser calories.

Light Turnip Curry

1 large cup chopped turnips
1 cup chopped turnip greens
½ teaspoon fenugreek seeds
1–2 slit green chillies
3 small tomatoes, grated
1–2 tablespoons desi ghee
A pinch of turmeric powder
Red chilli powder to taste
Salt to taste

- Parboil the turnips and keep them aside.
- Heat up the desi ghee and add the fenugreek seeds and slit green chillies.
- Cut the turnip into big chunks and add them to this oil. Stir-fry till they become slightly brown.
- Add 3 grated tomatoes. Cook till the colour becomes richer and the raw smell disappears. Add the turmeric powder, red chilli powder and salt to taste.
- Cook for a minute and then add some water till it reaches your desired consistency. Once the water starts boiling take it off the heat and then stir in the chopped greens.

20

INDIAN GOURDS

I really wish I had the palate I have now way back when I was a teenager. As a teen I loved my sugar and meat. I drank barely enough water and ate minimal amounts of vegetables. It is said that you can get away with poor eating habits when you are young. While you may be able to get away with it from a weight perspective, what happens inside is another story.

Poor habits continue with us to our twenties, and by then all the processed food, meats, refined flour and sugar would have already wreaked havoc on our hormones. These days every other girl has PCOD, PCOS, thyroid disorders or, like in my case, endometriosis. Food has such a deep impact, not just on our skin but also on our health and even our mood. So the truth is no, you can't get away with it. Eventually poor eating habits show up one way or another.

Now that I'm older I take good care of myself. So many foods that were once disgusting have become absolutely delicious for me. A case in point being Indian gourds, especially bottle gourd (*lauki*) and bitter gourd (karela).

I love their bland and bitter flavours, but more than that, I really enjoy how light and refreshing they make me feel after I've eaten them. I used to lack self-awareness, because of which I never observed how a food made me feel. Like most of us, I too was a slave to flavour and not the after-effects—the lightness, energy and digestibility that define good food.

When we only focus on stimulating our taste buds with high-salt, high-sugar foods, we naturally ignore the after-effects. Because these flavours are so stimulating for the tongue, we tend to get addicted and become numb to their effect on us. Blinded by intense flavours, we ignore the produce that is truly nourishing, not just for the skin or the body but also our minds. If clarity is the aim, we have to get rid of the foods that only appeal to our senses and learn to enjoy those that may not be so palatable. And slowly, as you eat better, your palate also changes. It's just a question of habit. Just like exercising makes us stronger, eating well reduces our cravings for processed, salty, sugary foods that offer no benefit except strong taste.

Bottle Gourd (Lauki)

I really started enjoying this vegetable a few years ago when I was undergoing treatment for endometriosis. It was summer and every day I'd drink a glass of lauki juice with one amla grated in. Despite the synthetic hormones I was on, my skin stayed clear. I have to credit this natural remedy for that. However one must take care to choose a gourd that is not bitter as that may be toxic. Lauki that is grown in unclean soil with polluted water can absorb toxins, which leads to the bitter flavour. So one must always taste it before juicing or cooking with it. A bland, almost sweet-tasting lauki is a wonderful and tremendously underestimated health tonic.

Science

It may not be glamorous but bottle gourd packs quite a punch. It's high in water content and contains vitamins C and B, along with soluble and insoluble fibres. A cup of lauki contains only 1 g of fat. This vegetable is highly beneficial for heart patients because the fibre practically sweeps cholesterol out of the body. Because of the fibre content, it's extremely good for gut health too. It increases haemoglobin, boosts energy levels, gets rid of impurities and mobilizes fat out of pockets where it's stuck in the body.

Bottle gourd is highly alkaline, immensely hydrating and supports the liver function. I've mentioned before and I'll say it again: a well-functioning liver is essential. If it is under stress or unclean, your body will not utilize any vitamins or minerals. Therefore, it's prudent to eat foods and develop habits that support and nourish this vital organ.

Tradition

In Ayurveda, bottle gourd is considered anti-inflammatory, which makes it excellent for skin diseases. It helps balance blood sugar levels, detoxify the blood and cool the body. It also works as a diuretic making it excellent for UTI. Traditionally, its juice is used for indigestion, acidity and ulcers. It is also considered to have sedative and antidepressant properties.

Therefore, as far as mind–body benefits are concerned, this vegetable works to give you clarity of not only the skin but also the mind.

Application

I enjoy a thin, watery bottle gourd curry with brown rice. It's my favourite summer food. It's light, yet filling, nourishing and energizing. One must eat according to the season—all gourds are refreshing during summer and must be enjoyed during the season. You can even use the water from boiling lauki to make a soup, which is excellent for weight loss.

Lauki is an excellent cooler. If you're suffering from heat rash or heat stroke, slice it and rub on the soles of your feet to soothe and cool the entire body. Heat rashes on the face can also be soothed by rubbing slices of raw bottle gourd on the skin.

Glow-Boosting Elixir

1 full bottle gourd
A few pinches of roasted cumin seeds
1 lemon
Rock salt to taste

- Juice the bottle gourd (taste it first to check for bitterness).
- Add the rock salt, cumin seeds and a squeeze of lime.
- Loaded with minerals, vitamins and antioxidants, this drink makes the skin healthier and shinier when consumed early in the morning.

Bitter Gourd (Karela)

Karela juice has always been the home remedy for acne. I don't know anybody who drank it when they were younger—I definitely didn't. But today, when I know so much about this glorious vegetable, I wish I had stomached its bitter juice. Also called bitter melon, it is an important element of one of the world's healthiest, indigenous food regimens— the Okinawan diet. Okinawa is a small island in Japan. Its citizens are among the longest living people in the world. Their food is low in fat and sugar and high in antioxidants. They especially love to eat bitter melon, with small amounts of meat and seafood.

Even in our country we know that the humble bitter gourd is extremely healthy. But knowledge is one thing and experience another. If you're suffering from acne or breakouts, it will transform your skin just by being a part of your diet.

Science

Bitter gourd helps diabetics immensely because it contains a substance (polypeptide-p) that works like insulin to bring down blood sugar levels. It also contains another compound called charantin which lowers these levels by improving glycogen synthesis in the liver. Glycogen is a molecule that is produced and stored in the liver when we eat more carbs than we require. When the sugar levels in our blood fall, this glycogen is broken down to release glucose into the bloodstream. Bitter gourd helps break down this glycogen and release it and thus it doesn't get stored in the body.

Karela is packed with vitamins A and C and various types of B vitamins. It also contains high amounts of folic acid (excellent for pregnant women), and flavonoids that help scavenge free radicals created by environmental toxins and stress. It's high in fibre, extremely low in cholesterol and is recommended for diabetics who want to balance blood sugar levels.

Tradition

Even in Ayurveda bitter gourd juice has been used to treat diabetes. In addition, this wonderful vegetable helps treat intestinal worms and liver disorders and enhance blood purification. It is traditionally prescribed for skin disorders and allergies, malaria and viral infections. Its bitter taste is a testament to its detoxifying and blood-purifying properties. Therefore bitter gourd is recommended to clarify the complexion.

Application

Cooking karela is an art. You have to add a bit of sweet and sour flavours to balance the bitter taste. The addition of caramelized onion adds sweetness and a dusting of raw mango powder over the cooked vegetable makes it delicious. You must really roast it well, because if it's a little watery, it won't taste good. My friend Varun Rana makes a crispy karela salad that makes a wonderful side or even a main dish if you want to eat light. Instead of frying the karela you can slowly dehydrate it in the oven to make it crispy and then toss it into a salad.

Of course you can always juice it—this is especially good for diabetics and also gives great results if you have acne. One word of warning: this vegetable can suddenly reduce blood sugar levels so it's better to juice it with other vegetables, especially if you have low blood pressure. If you're on a strict diet, avoid drinking bitter gourd juice. You need to eat a healthy, nourishing diet to support the function of this vegetable. Therefore it's always better to mix it with something more energizing—for instance, Indian gooseberry (amla), beetroot or carrot juice in winter and bottle gourd in summer. A great green juice recipe for summer would be 30 ml of fresh karela juice with lauki, cucumber, coriander, bell pepper, cumin powder and rock salt. Also, if you're drinking it first thing in the morning, keep a half an hour gap between the juice and any caffeinated or milky beverage.

Sweet and Tangy Stuffed Karela

5–6 karelas
2 big onions
2 teaspoons fennel powder
Red chilli powder to taste
Raw mango powder (*amchur*) to taste
2–3 tablespoons oil
Salt to taste

- Take the karela and slit lengthwise on one side.
- Fill a saucepan with water and 1 teaspoon salt. Boil the karelas in it for 5–7 minutes till they're light green. Pull them out of the water and set aside to cool.

- After 10 minutes pull out the seeds and flesh with a spoon and keep aside.
- Take the onions and slice them lengthwise. Fry them in a little bit of oil with salt. When golden, squeeze out the karela pulp and seeds and add them too. Stir-fry for a few minutes till soft.
- Add the fennel powder, salt, red chilli powder and raw mango powder to the onions. This is the stuffing for the karela.
- Stuff each of the karelas with the above mixture and tie with a string.
- Shallow-fry with a little bit of oil—when the karela is nicely browned, pull it out.
- This dish can last a couple of days because of the dried mango powder—a natural preservative.

21

GILOI

Guduchi, *amrita*, *giloi* or *giloy*, one of the most potent medicinal herbs of India, has seen a recent revival because of the unfortunate prevalence of mosquito-borne diseases. Dengue is one ailment that doesn't have a particular cure. But in small towns and villages people boil giloi with carom seeds (*ajwain*) and tulsi leaves to make a tonic that is said to prevent and reduce dengue fever. This is just one of the many uses of this powerful herb. A collection of studies published in 2012 showed that giloi extract has the ability to reduce tumour volume and prevent the side effects of radiation treatment.[1]

Science

In the medical world this herb is used for its potent, immunity-boosting properties. It's known to have anti-allergic qualities that make it an effective tool against hay fever. In fact, according to a study, it was found to have reduced 60–80 per cent of the symptoms of hay fever such

as a running nose, congestion, sneezing and nasal blockages.[2]
One of my favourite herbal remedies for the common cold is
Septillin. You have to take two tablets just when you feel like
you could be getting a cold. In my experience it really helps
halt the development of common cold or cough. The main
ingredient in this medicine is giloi.

This herb works by
stimulating the immune
system and increasing
the level of antibodies.
It is this property of
giloi that helps build
the body's resistance
against infections,
making it an
essential tool to fight
fevers and other diseases. While it is the stem of the plant
that is commonly used, each and every part has therapeutic
benefits. A decoction from its stem is used to treat skin
diseases and the leaves to cool a burning sensation, while the
whole plant is used to treat jaundice, diarrhoea and fever.
From the tips of its leaves down till its root, giloi is truly a
gift from nature.

This plant is a powerful adaptogen because it contains
phytoecdysteroids, chemicals that a plant creates to protect
itself from insects. The benefits of phytoecdysteroids include
improved protein synthesis and strength. The roots and stem
contain alkaloids that have anti-viral, anti-diabetic, anti-
inflammatory and anti-cancer properties. The glycosides
(also in the stem) help with neurological disorders. It contains

antiseptic compounds, and also helps improve liver function, which we know enhances skin condition. Studies have shown that not only does this herb control diabetes, it could also be as good as a standard drug for cholesterol. However, in conditions such as these, you must never replace your medicine without thoroughly consulting with your doctor.

Tradition

Guduchi is an ancient herb that finds mention even in old mythological texts. In the Ramayana, when Lord Rama wins the battle against Ravana, Lord Indra is very pleased and sprinkles nectar over the injured monkeys to bring them back to life. It is believed that the nectar that spilled on the earth gave birth to the giloi plant. 'Guduchi' literally means guarding the body from disease. The prabhava (power) of this herb is anti-toxicity, meaning that it clears toxins from the body.

It not only cleanses the body, but also rejuvenates and increases strength. It is said to promote longevity, work as an anti-ager and boost digestion and eyesight. It works on all the three doshas and helps build all the seven dhatus or tissues (plasma, blood, bone, marrow, muscle, bone and reproductive tissue) of the body. It is especially recommended in skin conditions related to pitta and vata. Therefore it works very well for inflammatory acne, burning sensations and rosacea, which are all pitta-related conditions, and dry, flaky skin, a sign of excess vata. It is the best immunomodulator, which is used to treat chronic conditions and a weakened immune system. Therefore it also works very well for any type of allergy. Because it stabilizes vata, which governs the nervous system, it helps soothe the mind and reduce irritability, thereby improving mood in general.

Giloi is revered not just in Ayurveda but also among the tribes of India who use it regularly to bring down fevers and infections. It is a creeper—when it grows on a neem tree its medicinal value becomes even higher. The vine grows wild in the jungles of India, Sri Lanka and Myanmar and doesn't require any special care. And yet, it has so much to offer.

In Ayurveda it goes beyond the medicinal value to a status that is sacred. In Vagbhata's *Ashtanga Hridayam*, it is referred to as *vakshagni dipani*, meaning it increases the light in the heart, thereby giving us the ability to withstand emotional challenges.

Application

You can take giloi powder or *sattva* with water, ghee, honey or milk, either once in the morning or twice in the day (morning and evening). If you opt for the powder, 6 g (a little more than 1 teaspoon) is the best dosage. When eating the sattva, reduce the dosage to about 2 g, which is less than ½ a teaspoon. For vata-related disorders, i.e., pain, irritability, dryness, joint issues and arthritis, mix it with 1 teaspoon ghee. In pitta-related skin conditions, like the ones mentioned earlier, eat it with a bit of mishri. And if you have kapha-related skin conditions (itching and oozing but not inflamed rashes), take it with 1 teaspoon honey. To boost immunity and improve health, just drink it with plain water or a cup of warm milk first thing in the morning.

If you have a fresh plant you can boil 4–5 leaves in a glass of water. Strain and drink it. Giloi is excellent to purify blood. It increases platelets, which is your personal army to fight infections. It can be taken in between meals but with a gap of about half an hour or 45 minutes.

22

WHEATGRASS

I usually begin my morning with 1 heaped teaspoon each of organic dried wheatgrass and moringa powders mixed in a glass of water with the juice of ½ a lemon and 1 teaspoon raw, organic honey. It's an alkalinizing, detoxifying, antioxidant rich drink that is perfect to begin the day. While I'd love to drink fresh wheatgrass juice, growing it can be a bit of a pain. The juice must only be extracted from freshly germinated seeds and the seeds can only be used once.

Thankfully we can always choose a dried powder, which is almost as potent as fresh juice. I say 'almost' because live plants have prana or the essential life force, while dried powders don't. But apart from that they contain all the other minerals and vitamins that are packed into fresh wheatgrass juice.

Science

This power-packed food contains vitamins A, C and incredible amounts of E, B6 and B12. It also contains huge amounts of other B vitamins that are essential for beautiful skin and hair such as thiamine, riboflavin, niacin and pantothenic acid. But that's not all. Just 4 g of fresh wheatgrass has almost half of your required daily allowance of iron, 85 per cent of copper and much more than your required daily amount of zinc and manganese. Zinc and copper help keep the skin clear and improve conditions such as acne and psoriasis. But more than anything else, wheatgrass contains chlorophyll, which is a potent antioxidant and anti-carcinogen. Chlorophyll also speeds up wound healing, aids liver function, removes heavy toxins from the body, reduces inflammation and increases haemoglobin. All this in a shot of juice or a spoonful of powder.

While no studies have proved that wheatgrass directly reduces toxicity in the body, it has been found effective in calming an inflamed colon (ulcerative colitis) and in reducing some harmful effects of chemotherapy. A study published in 2011 in *Functional Foods in Health and Disease* found that animals with low red blood cell counts, when given wheatgrass, had a healthy blood count level within five days.[1] Another 2004 study found that patients who had thalassaemia required fewer blood transfusions once they started consuming wheatgrass juice.[2]

Tradition

You may think of it as a global food, but wheat or barley grass was traditionally used in India during Navaratri. Called *khetri*, it's the symbol of fertility and was offered to the mother goddess on the ninth day of puja. The seeds are planted on the first day and by the ninth day you have fully formed grass. It's a beautiful reminder that what we reap is what we sow and shows that our ancestors probably already knew the benefits of this potent, health-giving grass.

Application

Fresh juice is always better than powder. If you want to grow your own grass get seven different pots where you can plant fresh seeds everyday so they're ready to be juiced by the seventh day. Always use fresh seeds for the next batch of wheatgrass.

If you're lazy like me, you can also mix 1–2 teaspoons of wheatgrass powder in a glass of water and drink it first thing in the morning. Combine wheatgrass juice with bitter gourd, cucumber, ginger and bell pepper juice for an energizing and detoxifying drink. Consume it first thing in the morning on an empty stomach.

23

MOONG

A few months ago I went on a cleanse to remove the toxins that one Ayurvedic doctor thought could be contributing to my endometriosis. Among a number of dietary tweaks, one was to not eat any beans or lentils other than moong.

Before I began this cleanse, moong dal was my least favourite. But after the cleanse, I prefer it over everything else. I don't avoid other lentils, but I've definitely become more conscious of how moong feels so light and grounding as compared to red beans, chickpeas or even *arhar* dal, which feels acidic and heavy. I don't suggest that you only eat moong dal. I just feel that it is far superior to others because it's so light, easily digestible and nourishing.

In my house moong is cooked every night for dinner—it is a staple ingredient, even if other dishes are on the table. My paternal grandfather who's in his 90s (and smokes like a chimney) eats moong dal with some greens every night.

Science

The speciality of moong dal and black chana (from which sattu is made) is that the bioavailability of nutrients is very high. So even if other beans or lentils have the same amount of nutrients, they will be absorbed much better by the body from moong or black chana. Foods that have high bioavailability don't cause stress to the body because it doesn't have to expend too much energy to digest and assimilate the vitamins and minerals present in them.

Moong is a nutritional powerhouse packed with vitamins C and K along with manganese, iron, folate and several other B vitamins. Just a cup of whole moong dal with peel contains 8–10 g of fibre. We only need 25–35 g of fibre a day. This wonderful lentil is extremely high in antioxidants and has about twelve phenolic acids that help improve the complexion by inhibiting common skin diseases. It also contains a variety of flavonoids that fight oxidative stress. Therefore moong helps neutralize the free radicals that destroy the body (and skin) at a cellular level. When you sprout anything you boost the vitamin and fibre content along with the bioavailability of nutrients. So sprouted moong is an excellent side or breakfast dish.

This dal also contains a moderate amount of protein (about 15 g per cup of cooked moong). However it must be mentioned that lentils are not a complete source of protein and must be eaten with grains such as rice to get all the nine essential amino acids. This is why our traditional dal–chawal is such a complete food.

Unlike other beans and lentils, cooked moong is extremely easy to digest and does not cause bloating. Perhaps this is the reason why yogis like to break their fast with washed moong dal that comes without the green peel. Though it may not have as much fibre or nutrients as whole moong, it is the lightest lentil in terms of digestion. Even when mothers wean infants off their milk, moong soup is one of the first baby foods given to them because it is bioavailable and easy to digest.

Tradition

Moong is also called *mudga*—one that brings joy and delight. In India we usually eat it in khichdi when we're recovering from an illness or trying to lose weight. According to Ayurveda, moong pacifies all the three doshas. It's sweet (nourishing), astringent (toning and detoxifying) and drying, which is why we always eat moong dal with ghee. It is purely sattvic in nature, and helps calm and balance the mind. Moong is a bit of an anomaly. Unlike other extremely nourishing foods that are usually heavy, this dal is nutrient-rich yet extremely light. It's known to enhance vision and concentration and works equally well whether eaten or applied.

Application

I find that when I eat moong dal cooked with lots of ginger, I feel very light and satisfied afterwards. The best part about it is that it is so delicious and versatile. You can make a dal out of it to eat with rice, drink it like soup, toss the sprouts into salads and also make moong dal chillas for breakfast (my favourite).

Traditionally moong powder is also used as a paste to clean your face, body and even hair. If you have a headache apply a paste made with moong flour and rose water on your forehead to soothe yourself. Wash after it is semi-dry. If you have tired eyes you can apply this same paste on your lids as a depuffing and cooling eye mask. Or you can simply mix its flour or paste with milk and use as a daily face and body cleanser. You can also grind soaked moong with marigold flower and milk to make a face mask to reduce blemishes.

Mix besan or moong dal powder, whole fat yoghurt (as much as you need to achieve a paste-like consistency), a spoonful of Manuka honey, a pinch of organic and good quality turmeric (to ensure that it doesn't contain any colour additives). Mix and apply on your face. Wash it off after 15 minutes. Lavanya Krishnan, the founder of the green beauty box service called The Boxwalla, also uses moong powder in place of soap on her newborn babies.

Exfoliating Moong Cleansing Powder

2 tablespoons moong dal flour
2 tablespoons barley flour
1 teaspoon orange peel powder
1 teaspoon almond meal
1 teaspoon neem powder
1 teaspoon sandalwood powder
A pinch of kasturi manjal or regular yellow turmeric
Enough oil, milk or rosewater to make a paste

- Mix the moong dal flour with barley flour, orange peel powder, almond meal, neem powder and sandalwood powder.

- Add a pinch of kasturi manjal or regular yellow turmeric to this.
- Depending on the season you can blend it with oil, milk or rosewater. For children or those with sensitive skin, milk works the best.
- You can make a big batch and store it but turmeric should be added right at the end just before mixing the paste.
- This is an excellent replacement for packaged cleansers and will help brighten and clarify the complexion.
- Do not use a physical exfoliant such as this if you are using acid toners or peel pads.

~

'Why is it that we do things which are not good for us? We assault ourselves with toxic food, agitated thoughts and hurtful actions, knowing fully well that they'll cause harm. We have the knowledge of what is right but just that isn't enough. Knowledge should translate into understanding and from there into acceptance and action. *Viveka* means discrimination and understanding what is good and not so good for me—this is what I call clarity. And it must be part of every aspect of your life. Think of your mind as a lake—if it's calm and clear, the reflection will be clean. If, however, the water is muddy and disturbed, even the reflection will be such. Clarity goes beyond just the quality of your complexion. It first begins with your thoughts and then reflects in your choices—clean food, clean living and, eventually, clear skin.'

—Kavita Khosa, founder, Purearth

~

PART III

RADIANCE

Succulent, elastic and lit from within, radiant skin is the ultimate symbol of health, happiness and love. We glow when we're filled with happy hormones. We shine when we take the time to look after ourselves. Indulging in self-care is seen as hedonistic by some, but for me it's a sign of love and self-respect. We often dismiss beauty rituals as too much work. But with a nourishing diet and adequate water, self-care has a multiplier effect. It enhances our skin, hair and general aura—it gives us an outward polish because we're satisfied from within.

People often tell me that they don't care about beauty. But that's a lie they're not just telling me but also themselves. Caring about outward appearance is seen as a shallow pursuit, and perhaps it is, if that's considered to be the only aspect of beauty. Being beautiful is not just about developing a pleasing appearance but also about building awareness of how foods, thoughts or people make us feel. We must choose only what makes us feel elevated.

I believe that we should be a little selfish and direct some kindness inwards so that we can give freely. When we're depressed we stop taking care of ourselves. So the need to improve appearance should be seen as a sign of a positive mind. Unfortunately, in today's world, we're surrounded by a fervour for the cosmetic aspects of beauty. We apply nine layers of skincare, wear make-up that looks like a mask and stock supplements to rival a doctor's cabinet. But that's not the self-care I'm talking about.

Looking after ourselves means choosing every element of our lives with care. We must be aware of what we eat, think and where we spend our time. When we eat and live mindlessly we disrespect our bodies, throwing in anything that catches our fancy. But when we really love ourselves, we take the time to pick the ideal option because we know we deserve the best. Still, it's impossible and perhaps even foolish to always choose health. Life is beautiful when lived in balance—wine with a nutritious dinner and chocolate afterwards is healthful and rewarding.

I've made Radiance the third part but it runs concurrently with Vitality and Clarity. Unlike some herbs in Clarity that must be consumed in small amounts, the foods listed in this part can be eaten in plenty by all. The speciality of these ingredients is that they're all packed with antioxidants. Poor skin is the result of free radicals or toxins attacking our cells. These harmful elements come from the environment or may be the result of a bad diet and stress. Antioxidants work like magnets, latching on to these toxins and vacuuming them out of our body.

Most glow-boosting foods can easily be a part of our everyday diet. We just have to build the awareness to include a few nourishing elements in every meal. To begin with, start noticing the different colours of fruits and vegetables, because each hue indicates a different antioxidant. So, the main rule for radiance is to eat the entire rainbow—the more colours we eat the more we'll glow. That, and a good night's sleep.

24

MORINGA

What surprises me most about nature is that it has so much to give and yet requires so little in return. Some of the most potent foods that heal and transform our lives need barely any food or water. Take aloe vera or giloi, for instance—they grow bountifully and provide us with so much without needing much care. Moringa is another really generous tree. It grows freely in the Indian subcontinent and seeks no special treatment. In fact, a few trees may even be on your way to work, but they're so understated that they could be unnoticeable. Today moringa is advertised as a superfood, which makes us forget its humble roots. It's the common drumstick or *sehjan* that we pull out of sambhar and keep on the side. For us it was just another tree until it was recognized for its phenomenal nutritional content.

Science

Every part of this miraculous tree is useful—from the roots to the flower, leaves and fruit. The best part is that it can withstand drought and mild frost, and is therefore extremely sustainable. It grows very easily and plentifully and does not require forests to be razed down for its plantation.

If you search on the Internet, you'll find that moringa has more than forty different antioxidants, more than ten times the calcium of milk, more than five times the vitamin C of oranges and more than ten times the vitamin A of carrots. It also contains twenty-five times more iron than spinach, fifteen times more potassium than bananas, about 25–30 per cent of your daily requirement of zinc, plus good amounts of phosphorus, magnesium and copper. All these numbers are correct, yet I must bring to your notice that they have been arrived at by comparing moringa to an equal volume of fruit or vegetable. So we're comparing a 100 g of moringa, which is extremely difficult to consume, with a 100 g of banana or carrot or spinach that we can eat very easily. That said, it is still one of the world's most nutrient-dense foods.

In many countries moringa powder is used to help children suffering from malnutrition restore their health. It is also given to new mothers to boost lactation. While the pods may not be as nutrient-dense as the leaves, they contain large amounts of vitamin C. The pods or the drumsticks are also packed with soluble and insoluble fibres that help improve gut health. In addition, the fruits, leaves and flowers contain amino acids that are the building blocks of muscular tissue. While a lot of greens lose their nutritional value after being processed, moringa's nutritional count increases when it is boiled or dried and crushed into a powder. Because of this reason, it can be preserved for a long period of time, without losing any nutrients.

Moringa powder proved its efficacy when it was used for a 2014 study with menopausal women. The women were given about 1 teaspoon (7 g) of the powder every day for three months. It was found that this significantly increased antioxidants such as superoxide dismutase, ascorbic acid and glutathione in their blood. There was also an increase in haemoglobin levels and a decrease in fasting blood sugar levels.[1] Because of its high nutritional content and its ability to scavenge free radicals and reduce inflammation, moringa is a precious and local glow-boosting food.

Tradition

Moringa is called the miracle tree or mother's best friend for good reason. In Ayurveda it is used to clean the liver, purify the blood and remove worms and acidic toxins. Its heating, pungent qualities make it penetrate tissues deeply and provide nutrition, while taking away impurities. Moringa also increases your digestive power. In Ayurveda, it is considered very beneficial for the eyes, which is not surprising when you consider its vast nutritional profile.

Application

I went for a face-mask masterclass conducted by Purearth, the green skincare brand, in Delhi. There, along with other clays and powders (bentonite, fuller's earth, neem, lavender, *gotu kola*, etc.), 1 teaspoon of moringa was also added to the mask because of its antioxidant benefits. Whether eaten or applied, antioxidants help repair and brighten the skin. According to Ayurveda, the paste of moringa leaves can be rubbed on the forehead if you have a headache or on burning skin. The oil extracted from its seeds is good for the complexion but is not suggested for acne and breakouts. Its bark can be made into a paste and applied on itchy skin, but not on an inflamed, breakout-prone complexion. So I prefer to eat rather than apply this miraculous herb.

I mix 1 teaspoon each of moringa and wheatgrass powders in a glass of water and drink it on an empty stomach first thing in the morning. It helps me begin the day on an alkaline note. The best thing about moringa is that it is easily available and generally safe for everyone to use. You can drink a fresh shot of juice from the leaves, mix the dry powder into water or a smoothie or add the drumsticks in sambhar to get a lot of fibre into your diet. Because of its high antioxidant content, anti-inflammatory properties and rich nutrient profile, moringa is a wonderful food to make the skin luminous from within.

25

INDIAN BERRIES

One of the best parts of going to school was visiting the *churan-wallah* during lunch break. He had sweet and savoury tamarind and pomegranate churans, candied ginger and, of course, bright red *ber*. I would eat everything with great relish till my tongue was raw, saving the delicious red berries to be enjoyed last. Before strawberries were grown in Mahabaleshwar and overpriced blueberries found their way into the Indian supermarket, there was ber (*jhar beri*), jamun (java plum), falsa (Indian sherbet berry), amla (gooseberry) and *rasbhari* (cape gooseberry)—delicious and medicinal Indian berries that are as good as their Western counterparts.

Today, it is difficult to find my favourite deep red ber that was earlier sold at every corner. The same goes for the *falsa*—another childhood favourite—that's now available only at a few stores. But these days even jamun—which we used to collect as it fell from the trees—comes packed in sterile plastic containers. Luckily, we still have amla because of its status as a health food. Rasbhari, which I hated immensely as a child, has also managed to survive.

A berry is a berry—just because blueberries are popular all over the world for their antioxidant content doesn't mean that our varieties are nutritionally inferior. They taste different from Western berries, which have a tart, fruity flavour. Our berries, while still sweet and tart, taste more earthy. I love this earthiness in our fruits, which makes them so versatile that they taste equally good in sweet and savoury dishes. You can dip them in honey or toss them in a salad with feta cheese. But it's not just taste that sets them apart; our berries are packed with immense medicinal benefits too.

Gooseberry (Amla)

My mother-in-law is one of those people who enjoys every season. She savours raw mangoes during summer, making a sweet and sour pickle with them using jaggery. She also makes a mint and coriander chutney with raw mango, salt and a couple of garlic pods. Come winter and amla is the raison d'être, and it replaces the raw mango in the delicious chutney, now with an added sprinkling of dried pomegranate powder.

Amla is the panacea of good health, and because of this reason, it is the most famous out of all our berries. People all over the world use it, especially to reduce the symptoms of type 2 diabetes. It helps reduce blood sugar, cholesterol and triglycerides. And, needless to say, because of its high vitamin C content, it also makes the skin glow from within.

Science

Just 100 ml of amla juice contains anything between 600–900 mg of vitamin C. Of course you never drink 100 ml of the juice, only a 30 ml shot. Indian gooseberry also contains iron that gets absorbed and assimilated by the body when combined with vitamin C. So in that sense, amla not only contains the best kind of nutrients but also in the most ideal combination.

The fruit is beautifying, restorative and health-giving because (other than spices) it's the most antioxidant-rich food in the world—much more than even goji, acai or blueberries. Amla also contains vitamin A, and small amounts of calcium, copper, manganese and phosphorus. Vitamin A is another powerful antioxidant which, together with these minerals, helps protect the skin and fortify the body.

The best part about amla is that the vitamins do not get destroyed when you juice, dry, cook, pickle or store it. Therefore it's a popular addition to Ayurvedic jams and powders, namely chyawanprash (where this is the main ingredient) and triphala (where this is one of the three ingredients). Amla's potent antibacterial, antioxidant and anti-inflammatory activities boost immunity and brighten your complexion.

Tradition

It is believed that amla takes care of you just like a mother does. It's *tridoshic*—works on all three doshas. Its cooling effect helps calm burning sensations in the eyes, feet and stomach. In fact, even premature greying, which is traditionally believed to be caused by excess heat, can be brought under control with the consumption of amla. It reduces hyperacidity, works like a cardiac tonic and also detoxifies the liver. Amla also cleans out impurities, improves eye health and helps slow down age-related wear and tear.

It has five tastes (sweet, sour, bitter, pungent and astringent), i.e. all except salty, and therefore holds all the therapeutic qualities of these flavours. So it nourishes the body, expels blockages, builds up immunity, removes infections and allergies and heals from within.

Application

The black colour of dried amla makes it extremely popular as an infusion in hair oil to keep the hair dark and shiny. My mother used to soak amla, *shikakai* (soap nut), and *rattanjot* (alkanet) overnight in a cast iron wok. This stinky mixture would be used to wash our hair as children. Both my brother and I were born with light brown curls, but my mother (like any other Indian woman) wanted her children's hair to be as black as the night. Weekly applications of brahmi amla oil and this amla-based wash really darkened our hair.

Gooseberries are also packed with pectin, the same fibre present in apples that helps clean our colon. Therefore it's a better idea to grate them into a smoothie, juice or chutney instead of drinking the juice. I eat organic chyawanprash all winter and firmly believe that it has strengthened my immunity. While amla is primarily a winter fruit, it is beneficial in summer too. A traditional preparation to eat during summer is an Ayurvedic jam called *amalaki rasayana*. It consists of amla pulp and juice. Unlike chyawanprash, which contains heating spices, this contains the fruit and nothing else. Therefore it's a good preparation even for diabetics who want to get the benefits of amla without the sugar. However, there are a lot of amalaki rasayanas in the market which contain sugar, so it's always wise to check the label before you buy it.

Amla helps boost immunity and health even in children. Those prone to asthma and bronchitis, or exposed to a lot of pollution, must drink 30 ml of fresh amla juice every day. If it gives you a sore throat then mix with another, less tart juice like that of bottle gourd. Though it tastes acidic, amla is extremely alkaline in nature. You can ferment and eat it as a pickle as fermentation of any fruit or vegetable increases its nutritional content. However, stay away from packaged juices as they contain added sugar.

Jamun and Falsa

A summer staple, these delicious deep-purple fruits have a more astringent taste as compared to blueberries. The dark purple colour of these berries reflects the presence of anthocyanins (the same antioxidant in blueberries and the bran of black rice). Both jamun and falsa help reduce heat in the body and are abundant during summer. As soon as the season begins we should eat a bowl of these berries every day.

Jamun

Come summer and
you find the ripe,
mouth-watering jamuns
lining the sidewalks. Monkeys and
parrots eat the berries straight off the
trees while we humans collect the ripe, heavy fruit
that falls on the ground. Eating this sweet, astringent and
sometimes tart berry brings back some cherished summer
memories. So jamun is definitely one of my most beloved fruits.

Science

Jamun is appreciated for its anti-diabetic effect on the body—
especially the seeds because they contain two compounds that
prevent the conversion of starch into sugar. Its astringent quality
really helps clean out the stomach. The best part is that it helps
burn fat without making you feel exhausted or burnt out.

The fruit is rich in antioxidants, iron, vitamins A and C,
along with trace amounts of other minerals and B vitamins.
The mix of potent antioxidants (flavonoids, phenolics,
carotenoids and vitamins) makes jamun anti-allergic, anti-
inflammatory, radio- and chemo-protective. It also fights
infections, increases haemoglobin, protects the heart and
shields the skin from pollutants.

Tradition

Mythology holds jamun in high regard because it is
considered to be one of the berries that Lord Rama ate during

his fourteen-year-long *vanvas*. Traditionally the fruit has been used to stimulate appetite, especially with a touch of black salt and pepper. Jamun's prabhava or special power is that it reduces excess sugar while nourishing the body. However, excessive amounts of jamun can lead to constipation because of its astringent qualities. Still, this astringency also makes it a wonderful wound healer. Jamun was considered the most important among all Indian berries so much so that in the old days India was called Jambudvipa—the place where jamun trees grow.

Application

Cooking destroys some of the antioxidants present in jamuns, therefore these berries are best eaten on their own or freshly juiced.

Clarifying Neem–Karela Powder

- Sun-dry the jamun and grind it. Mix it with equal parts of dried neem and karela powder.
- This is an excellent medicine to lower blood sugar levels.
- You can eat ½–1 teaspoon every day on an empty stomach or before you go to sleep. This also works as a mild laxative.

Falsa

I don't look at falsa as a fruit, but more as a savoury snack. I like to sprinkle black salt on it and add it as an unusual accompaniment to gourmet cheese. I love its crunchy seeds and pulpy outer layer. I enjoy it so much that every summer I make a falsa chutney by boiling the berries with a splash of water and a bit of salt, jaggery and roasted cumin seeds.

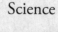

Science

Falsa contains anthocyanins, flavonoids and carotenoids, along with vitamins A and C—all of which work against environmental stress. Animal studies have shown that the leaves have anti-tumour qualities, while the fruit has radio- and liver-protective properties.[1] It is excellent for digestive health—just a fistful of this antioxidant-packed berry can reduce abdominal distress and bloating. It contains a lot of fibre so it's good for the gut and also helps reduce cholesterol.

Tradition

Falsa is a brilliant thirst quencher and does not dry the body like jamun. In ancient texts there are recipes for summer sherbets using falsa as it reduces excess heat. I like these fruits because they provide fibre for good digestion, antioxidants for improving skin condition and anti-inflammatory agents for soothing irritated complexions. Plus they are seasonal and local berries that are suited to our climate and genetics.

Application

Falsa sherbet is a common summer drink in many Indian households, especially because it reduces burning sensation in the skin and fever.

Cooling Falsa Infusion

1 tablespoon falsa berries
½ teaspoon raisins
½ teaspoon liquorice
½ teaspoon dates
½ teaspoon vetiver extract
Jaggery to taste

- Add all the ingredients, except jaggery, to a glass of water. Leave to infuse overnight.
- Strain, add a bit of jaggery and drink this infusion the next day.
- This drink is extremely cooling in the summer.
- This recipe is an alteration of the original *pancha saar panak* recipe from Vagbhata's *Ashtanga Hridayam*.

Jhar Beri

Also called *chanya manya bor*, these bright, squishy red berries are part of the buckthorn family. I do like the large greenish-yellow ber called Indian jujube, but these red berries are what childhood dreams are made of. They were found in the Ridge forests that surrounded our school in Delhi. These small shrubs would sometimes grow wild intertwined with the fences in the cantonment area where I lived. They were also found in front of most schools. So, for me, jhar beri is a reminder of those days when we'd spend afternoons picking and eating berries. But now I fear that my dearest berry lies forgotten. Something must be done to revive this beautiful and unique Indian fruit that's packed with vitamin C.

Science

Jhar beri prevents the formation of plaque in the arteries, improves digestion, reduces skin irritations and is especially good to boost immunity. It works on symptoms related to air pollution such as coughing and wheezing. The red colour is proof that it is high in antioxidants. It has sedative properties that help relieve anxiety and insomnia, and contains fibre to enhance digestion. It also helps regulate blood pressure.

Tradition

The berry finds a mention in the Ramayana in the story of Shabri, who tastes each ber for sweetness before giving it to Lord Rama. However, the cultivation of this ber has died over the last few years because it doesn't give as much pulp as compared to the large ber (Indian jujube), which actually is a Thai import.

Application

The best way to eat it is raw or pickled or as a preservative in *murabba*. Thankfully they're still relatively common in small towns and are available in large vegetable markets in big cities.

Rasbhari

Our humble rasbhari, swept aside for its supremely earthy flavour, lacks glamour because it is sold by street-side vendors. But did you know that this common berry actually comes from South America? Its scientific name is *Physalis peruviana* and it originated in Peru. I used to dislike its flavour as a child but as a grown-up I've learnt to really enjoy its rustic taste. I love that it can be used in both sweet and savoury dishes. It perks up a salad with its colour and flavour. Plus, the crunchiness of the seeds adds that extra bit of texture which goes beautifully with cheese. The best part is that it comes with a huge amount of nutrients.

Science

Rasbhari is one of those rare fruits that contain high amounts of vitamin K (usually found in green vegetables). It enhances heart, bone and skin health because it works as an antioxidant. Also known as golden berry, it contains small amounts of B vitamins and several other trace minerals including iron, copper and zinc (minerals essential for beautiful skin). They also contain double the amount of fibre present in apricots, goji berries, dates and prunes. Plus, they have the same amount of antioxidants as other fruits such as blueberries and raspberries, though the compounds are of a different kind.

The standout antioxidant of this marvellous berry is withanolide, which is also found in ashwagandha. Anolides are a group of compounds that are known for their anti-tumour, anti-inflammatory and liver-protecting properties. The berry's high beta-carotene content enhances eyesight and skin quality while its other immune-boosting, antioxidant properties help protect us against environmental assaults.

Tradition

Though this berry is native to South America, it has been in India for many decades. In folk medicine its fruit and leaves have been used to cure various ailments such as malaria and leukaemia. However, it is only recently that it is being celebrated as a gourmand's delight, in addition to being a health food.

Application

The yellow colour of this fruit—also called golden berry—is proof of its high beta-carotene content. Just a 100 g of rasbhari will give you 14 per cent of your daily requirement of vitamin A and about the same amount of vitamin C as an orange. Even the vitamin E content in the pulp of this berry is quite high. I prefer to eat these berries whole because of their huge fibre content. Fibre promotes good digestion, which is the first step towards beautiful skin.

Sea Buckthorn

My mother has been applying pure, wildcrafted sea buckthorn oil on her face for the last few months. After regular application her skin has become brighter, clearer and (I may be imagining it but) more lifted. I discovered the joys of sea buckthorn oil through Kavita Khosa, the founder of Purearth. And now I drink tea made with its fruit, eat supplements with its oil and even use a soap with its extracts.

Its miraculous benefits aren't so surprising when you just think about the characteristics of this plant. Sea buckthorn grows in the high altitudes of Ladakh, in the bitter cold, with minimum food and water. So it has developed the ability to not just protect itself but also thrive in the harshest of terrains. When we consume this berry we get the benefits of this robustness. Sea buckthorn protects us from environmental aggressors just the way it protects itself from the harsh climate in the Himalayas. Today, it is the buzzword in beauty, though till just a few years ago it was just another tart, undiscovered berry in Ladakh.

Science

The sea berry is one of the richest sources of vitamin C. Besides this, it has about fourteen vitamins including A, D, E, F, K, P and B complex. It also contains amino acids and powerful antioxidants such as anthocyanins, along with high amounts of minerals including potassium, calcium, magnesium, iron and phosphorus. They're one of the most nutrient-dense foods in the world—not only do they contain vitamins, minerals and antioxidants but also omega fatty acids. The berry has omega-3, 6 and 9, but its USP is that it is the richest source of the rare omega-7. A study conducted in 2014 by the Cleveland Clinic found that omega-7 showed substantial lipid- and inflammation-lowering properties when taken orally for just thirty days.[2] Because of this it also helps regulate blood sugar and fat, making it an effective tool against type 2 diabetes. However, take supplements with sea buckthorn only after consulting a doctor because it may interfere with your other medications.

Tradition

Commonly found in Jammu & Kashmir, Himachal Pradesh, Uttarakhand, Sikkim and Arunachal Pradesh, this berry is extremely sustainable. In fact, its potential was first explored when it was used for the afforestation of cold deserts in Ladakh in 1992. The tree only requires sunlight and can tolerate salty water and air. Because of its extensive root system it can bind even sandy soil very effectively, preventing erosion of mountains and waterbeds. It is naturally pest-resistant and therefore does not require pesticides. It is for these reasons that we first started exploring this berry outside of folk medicine where it was used to alleviate respiratory infections and boost digestion.

Application

Sea buckthorn oil is excellent to apply on the skin. The high vitamin C content makes the face look brighter, while its range of fatty acids adds lipids that add luminosity to your complexion. Unlike rose hip seed, which works well too but can cause breakouts, this can be used on (and will benefit) acne-prone skin. The oil contains salicylic acid, which makes up for 50–70 per cent of its phenolic content.[3] Salicylic acid is used as an acne remedy because of its ability to unclog and clear pores.

There's also gamma-linolenic acid (GLA) which acts like cement between cells, building up the skin's outmost layer called the barrier. When the barrier is strong, we are not very vulnerable to environmental aggressors because it acts like a shield. We are prone to fewer allergies, inflammation and breakouts. In fact, GLA is used in the treatment of atopic dermatitis. Sea buckthorn also contains linoleic acid (LA), which regulates sebum production, thereby making it suitable for acne-prone complexions. Because this oil contains beta-carotene, it offers mild protection from the sun. And the omega-7 speeds up healing of the skin. If I had to choose only one face oil, it would be sea buckthorn as it is immensely healing and versatile.

26

ROSE (DESI GULAB)

Rose is my favourite flower for many reasons—not just for its fragrance. I have typical pitta skin—it is rosy at its best and inflamed at its worst. So I keep rose water always at hand to mist my face and even spray into my eyes when I work for long hours on the computer. My grandmother—a great beauty who's not with us any more—used to say that rose water makes the eye whites so bright that they look almost blue. Even the taste of rose—so cooling and dry—soothes the stomach. So one of my favourite after-dinner indulgences is pan with gulkand (rose jam).

Rose is perhaps one of the most popular ingredients in skincare and fragrance. In the cosmetic section you'll find many 'rose' oils that are completely or mostly synthetic. Instead of calming your complexion, they cause breakouts. The price is a huge giveaway of how pure it really is. A few kilos of roses are required to produce just a millilitre of oil. So if it is cheap, well, it's not rose at all. If you want purity you have to buy it from a very reliable source and be prepared to pay for it. But don't use the essential oil directly on your skin.

Dilute it by adding it to a carrier oil like apricot or jojoba or mixing it in your regular moisturizer.

Then there's also poor quality rose water that is extracted using chemical solvents. While it will smell like rose, it has none of its benefits. Pure rose water should be steam-distilled, and this should be mentioned on the label.

Science

The bright red colour of our *desi gulab* is a testament of its high-antioxidant value. Just like other brightly coloured fruits and vegetables, rose is also a nutritious, edible plant. Its petals contain vitamin C, beta-carotene, B vitamins and vitamin K, along with antioxidants such as glycosides, flavonoids, anthocyanins and terpenes—all of which fight ageing by protecting the skin from environmental toxins. It's not just the petals but also the leaves of the rose that have therapeutic benefits. They contain both anthocyanins and chlorophyll that help scavenge free radicals, which cause ageing, and detoxify the body.

The most nutritionally rich part of the plant are its fruits—rose hips. They contain high amounts of vitamin A and C—ingredients that clarify and brighten the skin—because of which rose hip seed oil is highly revered in skincare. The wild harvested varieties can contain up to 40 per cent vitamin A, which gives the oil a slightly orange colour. However one must keep in mind that the vitamins in rose hip get destroyed in drying and processing, especially vitamins A and C. The most effective oils use a very fast, non-heating process such as supercritical CO_2 extraction that pulls out the fat without losing the nutrients. Look out for the method of extraction when you buy rose hip seed oil.

Tradition

The desi gulab or *rosa centifolia* is also called *shatpatri*—that which has a 100 petals—because the ideal rose is full and voluptuous. Another Sanskrit synonym of rose is *taruni* or beautiful young woman. According to Ayurveda, it is one of the varnya (skin-boosting) and *hridya* (heart-healing) ingredients. The light, cooling, easy-to-digest qualities of rose make it good for all the three doshas. However, it is especially good for pitta dosha, marked by red, reactive skin and a quick-to-anger temperament. Rose also helps nourish all the seven dhatus of the body—plasma, blood, muscle, marrow, bone, fat and reproductive tissue.

Traditionally rose was used to calm digestive disorders, in cases of heavy menstrual bleeding and to promote healthy elimination. Roses are highly anti-inflammatory, and are therefore beneficial in wound healing. They also have antibacterial, antiviral and antiseptic properties. Because of these qualities and the fact that they are packed with antioxidants, rose petals and rose water are excellent in face masks and creams. The fragrance of rose is said to be mood-lifting because it soothes the mind in the same way it calms the skin or the digestive system.

Application

Since rose is extremely cooling, 1 teaspoon of gulkand in a small cup of warm milk is an excellent remedy for people who suffer from body heat or inflamed skin. You can even use this remedy for constipation. You can consume up to 3 teaspoons of gulkand in a day to cool down the body. If you want to heal your gut you can eat 1 teaspoon of dried petal powder with 1 teaspoon of honey between meals with a 45-minute gap. You can also drink 20–40 ml of good quality rosewater between meals to hydrate your skin. To soothe tired eyes and reduce dark circles take a bowl of rosewater and add 10–15 drops of almond oil. Mix well. Soak two cotton pads in this mixture and keep it in the freezer for 30–40 minutes. Use these pads as an eye mask or, if you don't have the time, simply wipe the area around your eyes and go to sleep. Rose oil mixed with the paste of its petals and 1 teaspoon of fresh cream helps soften and awaken the dullest and driest of complexions.

You can also soak rose petals overnight in a tub of water. You'll find that there is oiliness on the surface of the water the next day. This is how rose essential oil is said to have been discovered in India by Noor Jehan. Use this water for a bath. Apart from scenting and hydrating your skin, it also controls sweat production. Lastly, to balance your emotions, take a few rose petals and a piece of pan leaf. Pound well in a mortar and pestle, strain and drink 4–5 drops of the juice every night before sleeping. This will help strengthen your heart.

Home-Made Rosewater

2 cups fragrant organic rose petals (the darker the better)
3 cups distilled water

- Pour the distilled water into a pan and add the rose petals.

- Over medium-to-high heat, bring the water to a boil. Then reduce the heat to a simmer till the petals lose their colour.
- Turn off the heat and steep the rose petals in the water for about 45 minutes till the water cools.
- Strain the rosewater (which will now be a beautiful pink colour) using a bowl and cheesecloth (or a fine mesh sieve).
- Discard the petals. The water can now be used to make a facial toner.
- To keep the rosewater from spoiling, store it in a glass bottle in the refrigerator.
- It can be kept for about two weeks.

Note: While this is a recipe for solvent-free rosewater, a good-quality steam-distilled variation will be more effective and therapeutic.

27

INDIAN GREENS

As humans we usually hate the things that are good for us. We replace lovely friends for the 'cool' crowd that isn't reliable. We work very hard to develop habits like smoking. And we choose bad boys over good men. It's only when we're older that we know how to treasure the good things—simple friends, nourishing habits and leafy greens—we turned away from when we were younger.

Eating greens is the most basic beauty habit you can develop after drinking enough water and getting a good night's sleep. Today, green powders, smoothies and juices have become immensely popular. While I do love all of the above, I also like to eat them in their traditional form—cooked in a subzi. Cooking with a bit of oil releases the oil-soluble vitamins and breaks down oxalic acid that prevents the absorption of certain nutrients from greens. I also believe that nutrition begins in the mouth. If you enjoy the taste of your food then naturally the benefits will be greater. Why eat something like it is medicine when you can add oils and spices to make it delicious?

Fenugreek (Methi)

A pungent winter saag, methi is a nutritional powerhouse. It contains vitamins A, B, C and K along with high amounts of iron, calcium, zinc and phosphorus.

Science

Methi reduces fevers, bronchitis and congestion, loosens excess mucus and lowers blood pressure. It also reduces abdominal discomfort, works as an antibacterial, anti-ulcer, anti-helminthic (worm) agent, protects the digestive system and the liver and also provides a huge boost of antioxidants.

Tradition

Cooking does not destroy the minerals in methi, which is one of the oldest medicinal herbs known to man. In Ayurveda, the plant is called *methika*—that which improves the intellect. It is light, oily, nourishing, warming, bitter and pungent. It helps detoxify the body by purifying the blood. According to ancient texts it is good for horses because it is very strengthening. Because of this, it is also called *ashwabala*—strengthener of horses. Traditionally the leaves were used to improve digestion, haemoglobin levels, hair and skin quality.

Green superpower: Methi can reduce blood sugar, which makes it perfect for diabetics.

Mustard (Sarson)

Mustard comes in the same family of cruciferous vegetables such as collard and kale. It contains high amounts of vitamins A, C, E and K along with iron and calcium.

Science

The vitamins and minerals in mustard prevent osteoporosis, improve eyesight, clarify the complexion by preventing acne, reduce inflammation in the body and boost immunity. The real strength of this green lies in sulphur-based compounds called isothiocyanates which help detoxify our bodies on a cellular level. Mustard leaves are also high in fibre and chlorophyll. Because of these two elements they remove environmental toxins from the bloodstream and improve gut health.

Tradition

According to Ayurveda, mustard leaves are pungent, heavy and drying. They have the tendency to trigger acidity because of which they're never cooked on their own and are always consumed with other greens to take away their 'burning' effect. Plus they must be consumed only when they're in season, i.e. during winter.

Green superpower: Mustard leaves are very strengthening
and therefore perfect for athletes, new mothers and
pregnant women.

Mom's Mustard Saag

750 g mustard leaves
200 g *bathua* (lamb quarters)
200 g spinach
2 whole garlic, chopped
2 small handfuls of chopped ginger
1 tablespoon coarsely ground bajra
1 tablespoon coarsely ground corn flour (*makki atta*)
4–5 tablespoons ghee
2–3 medium tomatoes
A pinch of asafoetida
Red chilli powder to taste
Salt to taste

- Wash the mustard leaves, bathua and spinach. Chop
  finely.
- Place them in the pressure cooker.
- Now add 1 whole garlic and 1 handful of ginger and top
  it up with the bajra.
- Add 2 glasses of water, close the pressure cooker and
  cook on low flame after the first whistle for an hour
  and a half.
- Once cooked, open the cooker and lightly pound the saag
  till it becomes thick and almost creamy. Let it remain on
  low heat.

- Mix the makki atta with water to make a paste. Add it to the saag, while stirring continuously. Let it cook for 5–10 minutes. Also add salt.
- Then in a small wok on the side, heat the ghee.
- When hot, add a pinch of asafoetida. Then stir in the remaining chopped garlic and ginger.
- When they're golden brown, add a little red chilli powder to taste and 2–3 medium sized tomatoes.
- When they're soft, temper the saag with this mixture and cover immediately. Keep it covered for five minutes.
- Enjoy with rotis and more ghee.

Purslane (Kulfa)

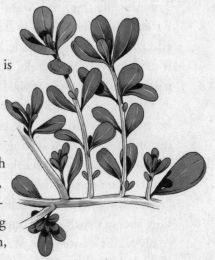

Purslane, pigweed or *kulfa* is actually a succulent and not a leaf. While it isn't so popular on our kitchen tables, it is widely used as a medicinal plant. It comes packed with nutrients including vitamin A, B-complex, vitamin E, beta-carotene and vitamin C, along with zinc, copper, calcium, magnesium and calcium.

Science

Interestingly, unlike other greens, kulfa contains a precursor (alpha-linolenic acid or ALA) to omega-3 fatty acids that is mostly found in fish. It is also the richest source of gamma-linolenic acid (GLA) among green vegetables. GLA helps improve skin conditions such as psoriasis and eczema. It also contains slippery mucilage that aids healthy elimination. The best part is that it grows as easily as a weed and doesn't require much care. It's so healing and nourishing that it's the main ingredient in some of the most expensive skincare products in the world.

Tradition

Traditionally this green was used to strengthen the digestive system, detoxify the body and hasten wound healing. Its effect on the body is rajasic, which means it is energizing. It's also cooling and works as a diuretic. In the olden days a paste of its leaves was applied to burns and scabs because of its refrigerant and healing properties. Since it has a cooling effect, kulfa must only be eaten in summer when it's in season. It has a slightly tangy taste, which makes it a great addition to salads, especially in Indian summer when leafy greens aren't so abundant.

Green superpower: Kulfa is especially good to control skin allergies such as urticaria and rashes. Allergies are the result of one's antibodies overreacting to a perceived danger. Kulfa helps reduce this reaction.

Medicinal Summer Saag

500 g kulfa leaves
2–3 tablespoons mustard oil

1 teaspoon cumin seeds
1 medium onion
Turmeric
Salt to taste

- Pour the mustard oil in a pan and heat it till it burns and smokes.
- Add the cumin seeds and the onion chopped lengthwise.
- Then add the clean kulfa leaves with salt and turmeric and fry till it is cooked well.
- Enjoy with plain rice.

Amaranth (Chaulai)

Amaranth seeds (like quinoa, this is also not a grain) are loved all over the world because they're highly anti-inflammatory. I love the laddus made with amaranth and jaggery. And its greens are as nutritious as the seeds.

Science

Did you know that amaranth leaves are one of the richest sources of vitamin C? And that they contain the highest amount of vitamin K among edible greens? Vitamin K is essential in strengthening the bones and preventing nerve damage. It also helps speed up wound healing and reduces bruises, dark circles, spider veins, redness and inflammation. The leaves also provide you with beta-carotene, B vitamins, zinc, copper, manganese and calcium. In addition, they're also one of the best sources of plant protein available in India.

Tradition

According to Ayurveda, amaranth leaves are sweet and nourishing. They reduce dryness and therefore are recommended for arthritis. They are laxative, diuretic and help bring down inflammation. Amaranth leaves reduce burning sensations and are therefore beneficial in skin problems such as inflammatory acne. You can either drink the juice or saute the leaves with mustard seeds and garlic.

Green superpower: Amaranth leaves are good for increasing the haemoglobin level and blood count. They're also strengthening, and are thus good for those who are anaemic. While mustard leaves strengthen the bones, amaranth leaves fortify the blood.

Lambs Quarters (Bathua)

This ancient weed grows wild, requires no care and still has so much to give. A small portion of bathua leaves gives you more than your daily requirement of vitamin A, half the amount of vitamin C and a quarter amount of calcium.

Science

Bathua leaves are an excellent form of protein. In fact, greens generally give more protein than other vegetables. In addition, it is one of those rare plants that has a balanced amino acid profile usually found only in animal protein. One of the amino acids it contains is lysine, which is found in very small amounts in plant foods.

However, bathua is high in oxalic acid, which inhibits the absorption of certain nutrients. Cooking breaks down this acid, because of which it is always better to eat these leaves in a cooked subzi, soup or wrapped in paranthas (my favourite). It is important to understand that all leafy greens give you a heavy dose of minerals and may not suit everyone, especially those with kidney stones. So it is better to cook them to make these minerals more digestible instead of eating them raw or adding them to smoothies. Cooking the greens with a bit of oil also helps with the absorption of vitamins A and K. When you eat them with a grain like rice or roti, you are able to utilize all the nutrients in them in a much better manner.

Tradition

Traditionally, bathua leaves were used in deworming and antimicrobial treatments. It is considered to be a potent detoxifier and its juice helps to improve liver and kidney function and reduce urinary infections.

Green superpower: Bathua leaves purify the blood, increase haemoglobin and boost heart health.

Mom's Bathua Raita

1½ cups bathua leaves

2 cups yoghurt
1 teaspoon roasted cumin seeds
Salt to taste

- Boil the washed, cleaned and chopped bathua leaves.
- Squeeze out the excess water.
- Add the leaves into beaten yoghurt. Then add the salt and roasted cumin seeds.

28

INDIAN SEEDS

When we think of seeds, our mind usually goes to varieties like pumpkin and sunflower. Don't get me wrong; I love those seeds. Flax and sesame too. They're high in essential fatty acids, vitamins and minerals, plus add delicious texture to any dish. But here I'm talking about the seeds of our spices that are low in calories and high in antioxidants.

Our traditional Indian diet is extremely balanced. We regularly add these seeds to our dishes, but they can also be consumed on their own for therapeutic purposes. You can grind them to make a health powder or boil or soak them in water to create an infusion.

Most of the benefits I talk about in this chapter are common knowledge. Your grandmother may not be surprised by these facts, but perhaps they will change your life. Indian food is extremely flavourful. Interestingly, we have achieved these flavours by adding medicinal foods and not unhealthy ingredients such as white flour and cheese. Seeds add immense taste and come with healing properties. So instead of just using them in traditional recipes you can experiment with them too. Why not use an oil infused with the traditional five-seed panchphoran in a salad or grilled chicken? Or temper some jeera to mix into buckwheat pancakes?

Our seeds are extremely versatile and unique tasting, and their benefits will completely blow your mind. But you must keep in mind that spice seeds contain volatile oils and therefore must be consumed in small quantities only.

Fennel (Saunf)

Let's begin by setting the record straight. Aniseed is the small saunf and fennel is the big saunf that we use in cooking. They come from different plants but are part of the same family called apiaceae. Both have that delicious liquorice-y flavour because of which saunf is so popular as a mouth freshener.

Science

The benefits of eating aniseed after meals go beyond its cosmetic, mouth-freshening effect. Both aniseed and fennel contain a volatile oil called anethole that has been shown to reduce inflammatory gum disease in animal studies. The same anti-inflammatory action makes it an effective tool against nausea, indigestion, cramps and gastric discomfort. Both fennel and anise also have expectorant action, meaning they help clear phlegm and mucus. In addition, they're a good source of B vitamins, vitamin C, manganese, copper and fibre.

Tradition

Saunf is excellent for pitta personalities, who have reddish, rosy complexions. It is light, oily, nourishing and pungent. Therefore it increases digestive fire. When consumed before a meal it acts as an appetizer and after a meal it works as a digestive. It is extremely cooling and can be eaten and applied. Because of this reason you'll find that powdered saunf is an addition to many ubtans (cleansing powders). It detoxifies the body with its diuretic action and also helps increase milk production in new mothers. It is a completely sattvic food and therefore helps calm and balance the mind.

Application

I became interested in fennel as a great ingredient after I saw the founder of one of India's biggest beauty brands with skin that was extremely clear and radiant. He told me that the secret to it was fennel water which he drank on an empty stomach every morning. Traditionally, saunf was used to reduce burning sensations in the body, which as we know reflects its anti-inflammatory benefits. If you have red, reactive, rosacea-prone skin, then a small dose of fennel or an infusion in water will help soothe your complexion.

Fennel seeds are also suggested as an analgesic, especially to reduce period pain. They clear worms and microbes, relieve constipation, improve strength and immunity and also work as a cardiac tonic (as the fibre helps reduce cholesterol). You can infuse ½ a teaspoon of fennel seeds in a cup of hot water and drink it after meals. Or you can soak them in warm water overnight and drink that first thing in the morning.

Carom (Ajwain)

Carom seeds or ajwain is used in most Indian homes in food and home remedies—be it for period pain or indigestion. My mother makes suji halwa with carom seeds and dry fruits in winter because it is extremely warming and improves flow during menstruation. My grandmother says that it helps with digestive issues. It's not a surprise then that it is added to fried foods such as paranthas and pooris that could otherwise cause indigestion.

Science

Carom seeds contain calcium, iron, phosphorus and some B vitamins, but the active ingredient is a volatile oil called thymol. Responsible for its thyme-like taste, thymol has been shown to have antifungal and antimicrobial properties. Because of this reason it helps reduce candida fungus in the gut. We get candida overgrowth when we take too many antibiotics, oral contraceptives or are on a diet high in refined carbs, sugar and alcohol. The signs include migraine, brain fog, inflamed, breakout-prone skin, mood swings and digestive issues. Ajwain extract has proved to be effective in breaking down this fungus which can release toxic by-products into your bloodstream.[1]

Tradition

Ajwain helps improve breathing, reduces inflammation, neutralizes free radicals from environmental toxins and improves digestion. It has liver- and kidney-protective properties, because of which it is a potent detoxifier. Carom seeds are hot, dry and light. So while they help reduce abdominal cramps, they also increase burning sensations, because of which they should not be consumed as a pure infusion or decoction by people with pitta dosha. Because of their warming nature, they are used extensively to reduce period pain.

Application

Carom seeds are especially good for people with polycystic ovarian syndrome (PCOS). Besides relieving menstrual cramps, they help reduce bloating too.

Ajwain Period Pain Reliever

2 teaspoons carom seeds
1 teaspoon jaggery

- Boil a little more than a glass of water with the carom seeds and jaggery.
- Let it boil for a few minutes.
- Drink it hot to relieve menstrual cramps.
- If you want to use this recipe to improve digestion (or if you feel hot very easily), use only 1 teaspoon of the seeds.

Fenugreek (Methi)

I know two women with extremely beautiful skin, and both eat fenugreek seeds every morning on an empty stomach. One of them is a Middle-Eastern beauty blogger and the other is my yoga guru, Seema Sondhi. A lot of Indians eat fenugreek powder with a bit of water on the side on an empty stomach in the morning. This has been shown to reduce cholesterol and balance blood sugar levels. Therefore these seeds are especially popular among people with diabetes and heart disease. Fenugreek is immensely beneficial for skin and hair too.

Science

When infused into hair oil, it helps stimulate hair growth and prevents greying. It can also be considered a skin food because it comes packed with B vitamins such as folates, along with vitamins A and C and skin-benefitting minerals like copper, zinc, iron and selenium. Fenugreek seeds also help the skin by clearing the lymphatic system of toxins and thereby helping it function better. Our lymphatic system helps drain out wastes from the body and if it isn't functioning properly, it can lead to dull, acne-prone, irritated skin.

One animal study showed that fenugreek increases the growth hormone by stimulating the pituitary gland.[2] Another 2015 study[3] found that its compound diosgenin (a saponin) is effective in treating metabolic disease, which is a cluster of conditions including high blood pressure and sugar, fat around the waist and increased triglyceride levels. The same saponin, being a phytoestrogen (plant oestrogen), is considered a natural alternative to hormone replacement therapy, especially for postmenopausal women.

Tradition

Traditionally, fenugreek was used to reduce bloating, digestive problems and abdominal pain. It is considered highly beneficial for the skin and hair. It purifies the blood, improves liver function, induces sweating and is also considered to be a tonic for the nerves. In Ayurveda, the leaves are considered cooling for the body, while the seeds are warming. Therefore, if you are a pitta type (burning eyes, red, irritable skin), you must take this as a supplement only after consulting an Ayurvedic doctor. Another thing to note is that when you take fenugreek powder as a supplement it can become a part of your body odour. So try to observe the effect it has on your body before making it an integral part of your diet.

Application

There are so many ways to eat these beautifying seeds. You can soak 1 teaspoon of methi seeds in half a cup of water and have it first thing in the morning. You can also make a powder with flax, ajwain and jeera in the same ratio, and half the quantity of methi seeds (20:20:20:10). Eat 1 teaspoon of this powder before you go to sleep to help burn fat and lower cholesterol.

Methi Bhringraj Hair Oil

200 ml sesame seed oil
¼ cup fenugreek seeds
¼ cup dried *bhringraj*
¼ cup amla

- Heat the sesame seed oil in a pan.
- Add the fenugreek seeds, dried bhringraj and amla.
- Boil for 5 minutes and then simmer for 15–20 minutes.
- Allow to cool and then strain the oil in a clean jar.
- Massage on scalp and hair once a week. Leave overnight for best results.
- Fenugreek seeds have been praised in Ayurveda for treating many hair problems like premature greying, excessive hair loss and dandruff. This oil stimulates hair growth and strengthens hair follicles. Its antifungal and antimicrobial properties also help clear scalp infections.

Coriander (Dhania)

It's interesting to see how herbs and their seeds calm down inflammation in the body. Plant foods are packed with antioxidants that fight free radicals and prevent damage. For these reasons they help fight and prevent chronic disease. Even herbs as humble as the coriander help fight diabetes, reduce cholesterol and improve digestion. In our country, coriander is perhaps the most common ingredient used in cooking. We make chutneys with the herb, use it as a garnish and add the powdered seeds to curries to thicken it. We use it in most of our dishes, without actually understanding how beneficial it really is.

Science

Both the seeds and leaves contain antibacterial components (aliphatic [2E]-alkenals, alkanals, dodecenal) that make coriander a natural food preservative. It's especially good at getting rid of food-borne bacteria, which makes me think how amazing it is that our ancestors made this herb a part of our daily diet. Coriander seeds are also great at building bones because they contain good amounts of calcium and phosphorus. They also have huge amounts of vitamin C along with skin-benefiting B vitamins, copper and zinc. More than 40 per cent of coriander seeds is insoluble fibre—it serves as food for all the good bacteria in the gut, sweeps out cholesterol and increases bulk in the stool for better elimination. I'm of the firm belief that good digestion is the way to clear, radiant skin. Often we don't eat enough fibre and drink adequate water. The best way to increase fibre intake is not through supplements, but via fresh vegetables, fruit and seeds.

Tradition

According to Ayurveda, coriander leaves are cooling and the seeds a bit warming. They help balance all the three doshas and work as a detoxifier and diuretic. The seeds and leaves are especially beneficial for the stomach and bladder. In fact, they help stimulate appetite by rekindling the digestive agni without creating acidity. They relax the mind, calm the body and boost immunity, while the juice of the leaves reduces allergies and urticaria.

Application

The great thing about coriander is that both the leaves and seeds have a vast antioxidant profile. They contain several volatile oils, flavonoids and polyphenols—all of which help neutralize molecules that damage cellular structure. I once met a woman who was in her seventies but had the most even-toned, wrinkle-free skin. She told me her secret was drinking coriander water. She just boiled a handful of coriander leaves and drank the tea. However, coriander leaf water is so cooling that it must not be consumed by people who have painful joints as it can worsen the pain.

A few years ago, when I was struggling to lose weight, my nutritionist made me drink two glasses of coriander water in the morning. Of course I followed her diet and cut out a lot of sugar and fattening foods from my diet, but those glasses really made me feel like I began my day by detoxifying from within.

To make an infusion, soak 1 teaspoon of coriander leaves in warm water overnight. Drink on an empty stomach first thing in the morning to detoxify the body, get rid of water retention and reduce hypertension. Eat the seeds for their fibre content.

29

MARIGOLD (GENDA)

All through my twenties and most of my thirties I've been a pitta-dominated person. What this means is that I am prone to redness, which on a good day can look rosy and on bad days, angry and blotchy. Most women consider a blush the most transformational tool in their make-up kits. But I've never owned a single blush in my life because it just makes me look like I have a rash on my face.

A good skin day for me is when it looks more yellow than red, because that's when I know that my skin is feeling calm. I choose beauty ingredients for their powers to pacify my skin and one of the most powerful pacifiers is marigold.

As is the case with people, some of the most enriching plants are often the humblest. Our own *desi genda*, one of my favourite flowers, may not have any romantic stories attached to it like the rose, but it sure packs a punch. I used marigold-infused water as a toner and found that it really helped calm my complexion, especially on days when I hadn't slept much. Its bright orange colour is proof of its high antioxidant profile. If we choose brightly coloured fruits and vegetables,

why not flowers? You can infuse its petals in oil, boil it in
water for a tea or add it to rosewater to make it more effective
and soothing. I love this flower because it really feels like a
balm on my skin—calming, healing and soothing.

Science

Like any bright orange fruit or vegetable (orange, carrot,
pumpkin) marigold is also rich in carotenoids. Indian
marigold is especially high in a carotenoid called lutein,
which is related to vitamin A and beta-carotene. Lutein
is known for its ability to reduce oxidative stress caused
by environmental factors and lifestyle, thereby reducing
inflammation in the body. For this reason it can prevent age-
related decline of eyes and cardio-metabolic issues such as
heart problems and diabetes.

Marigolds also contain two potent flavonoids
(patuletin and patulitrin), which work as antibacterial
and anti-inflammatory agents. In addition, the roots of
the tagetes species (from which marigold comes) are rich
in alpha-terthienyl, a plant metabolite that gets activated
when exposed to UV light. This metabolite works to
reduce disease-causing microbes, such as bacteria, fungi,
insects and some viruses. Marigold flowers are also highly
nutritious and other than carotenoids and flavonoids,
also contain vitamin C, which is one of the most
powerful antioxidants.

A 2018 study published in the journal *Toxicological
Research* found that marigold extract does have significant anti-
ageing potential. Because it has a high level of polyphenols, it

helps collagen production and reduces damage to skin cells.[1] This, along with its soothing, anti-inflammatory properties, makes it the unsung hero of glowing skin.

Tradition

The main tastes of marigold are bitter and astringent, both of which are cooling for the body. The petals can be used to make cooling infusions, the paste of the leaves can be applied on breakouts, while its juice works as a diuretic. You can boil the dry leaves and petals to make a detoxifying tea or crush them to extract juice that can be used directly on the skin or mixed into a face pack.

I personally find that anything rich in antioxidants, especially vitamin C, can be applied on the skin to brighten and even out the skin tone. The only exception that I would make are citrus fruits, which I find too acidic for topical application. Also, the vitamin C from citrus fruit degrades very rapidly when exposed to light. Therefore, it is not very effective.

Application

Interestingly, there's a reason why we use strings of marigold flowers for decoration. It's because they keep bugs out of the house. Marigold is antimicrobial and antiseptic, because of which it is widely used in cleansers and skin creams. The juice of its leaves and flowers helps heal wounds and also cools down the skin. You can also add the petals to summer salads for an interesting flavour.

Glow-Boosting Anti-Acne Mask

5 marigold petals
1 teaspoon sandalwood powder
1 teaspoon freshly ground tulsi

- Grind all the ingredients together and make a paste.
- Apply on clean skin, leave it on for 10 minutes and then wash off.

30

BITTER APRICOTS

As I grow older and my skin becomes drier, I look for oils to enhance the barrier of the outermost, protective layer of my skin. I've struggled with acne growing up. Anyone who has had to deal with breakouts knows that most of the products in an anti-acne regimen are drying and astringent in nature. Soapy, medicated face washes, harsh anti-acne creams, peel pads loaded with alpha- and beta-hydroxy acids—all strip the skin of our precious barrier, which is mainly made up of oils. The irony is that the more we strip this barrier, the more sensitive our skin becomes to pollutants because the natural shield is gone. The skin becomes thinner, redder and reactive. In fact, the same thing happens when we use prescription-strength retinol. I know it's touted as the best wrinkle remover, but it burnt my skin when I used it every day.

But I digress. Bitter apricot oil, when compared to almond and even coconut oil, is extremely light and gets absorbed quickly. I've used it even in the hottest summer days to massage my face and have never faced a problem.

I use it on my body in winter when the skin becomes dry and itchy. I find it works better than any expensive body lotion. I massage it in as a hair oil and even use a couple of drops as a hair serum for the smoothest, shiniest strands. But these are merely just the cosmetic benefits of this wonderful ingredient that goes way beyond just giving you beautiful skin.

Science

Bitter apricots contain laetrile (also called vitamin B17 or amygdalin) because of which it is both popular and notorious. One part of laetrile is cyanide which, according to folklore, selectively kills cancer cells. But while there is empirical evidence to suggest it may work, there are no human studies to prove the same.

Some people consider these fruits to be poisonous because of the cyanide content. However, one must keep in mind that anything extremely therapeutic can also be toxic—it just depends on the quantity. In very high amounts even water can be extremely toxic. The same goes for cyanide in fruits— it just depends on how much you're eating. Even apple seeds and bitter almonds have cyanide in them. But in limited quantities, they are not fatal.

In terms of application, there is conclusive proof that bitter apricot oil can work on inflammatory skin conditions such as eczema and psoriasis. In people with psoriasis, the skin cells go into overdrive by multiplying themselves five times faster than normal, resulting in dry flakes. Research has shown that bitter apricot essential oil actually stimulates the breakdown of these extra skin cells (keratinocytes), thereby providing relief from the condition.[1]

Long-term consumption of bitter apricot kernels has also been shown to reduce cholesterol in the body, making it a wonderful tool to fight cardiovascular disease. The kernels also contain another interesting compound called pangamic acid (also known as vitamin B15) which increases endurance and promotes oxygenation of vital organs. Vitamin B15 was also earlier considered in the treatment of cancer. Both these so-called 'B vitamins' are considered unsafe for consumption now in the US, which increases the intrigue around this food that many consider a potent nutraceutical.

Tradition

In Ayurveda, bitter apricot oil is recommended only for topical purposes. However, these kernels are an important staple of the diet of people living in the Hunza valley in Pakistan, who are one of the world's healthiest, longest-living people. It is assumed by many that the reason the Hunzas lead long, disease-free lives is because they consume a lot of bitter apricot kernels. Even in Kashmir and Ladakh, bitter apricot oil is used extensively to enrich the complexion and relieve dryness.

Application

Bitter apricot oil is a boon for skin diseases and is used in many treatments as it is light and gets absorbed quickly. I like to add bitter apricot oil instead of coconut oil to enrich raw cacao energy balls as it has a unique taste. I also drink it often. Even when applied, it is enormously soothing and beneficial. Bitter apricot oil is an excellent pain reliever, especially for people suffering from arthritis. Half a teaspoon of this oil is safe to drink every day.

Kashmiri Skin Balm

½ cup shea butter
3 tablespoons aloe vera gel
5–6 drops apricot oil
2–3 tablespoons raw honey
2–3 tablespoons rose water

- Melt the shea butter in a double boiler. Once it melts, add the aloe vera gel, apricot oil, raw honey and rosewater and mix till you get a creamy consistency.
- Keep the mixture in the fridge for about 15–20 minutes.
- Take it out of the fridge after it has cooled down.
- Using a hand mixer, whip it till it is light and fluffy.
- Refrigerate the cream and use when required as a night cream.
- It works well on extremely dry skin.

Home-Made Apricot Body Wash

- Take 3 parts unscented liquid Castile soap mix.
- Add 1 part honey and 1 part apricot oil.
- Pour all the ingredients into a clean glass container and shake to mix them well.

- Do not fill the jar up to the top as it needs air to mix as well as bubble up. The ingredients will separate again when left to stand for a while but that doesn't matter. Just give it a good shake when you have to use it.
- This body wash is great to moisturize and clean your skin.

~

'About twenty years ago we were driving to Rishikesh. It was almost dusk when we saw a group of 8–10 men in saffron robes. Among them was one man who was the most radiant person I've ever seen. There was so much light in his face that even after twenty years all of us remember him clearly. He was a sadhu coming out after a long *sadhna*—for months or years, I don't know. We found out later that at that time he was 101 years old, but he looked no older than twenty-five. Radiance for me is an outward manifestation of bliss. It comes from living in harmony with nature—of living, eating and sleeping well. It's a state of complete balance and contentment. Most people think that being beautiful will make them happy, when actually it's the other way round—being happy makes you radiant.'

—Mira Kulkarni, founder, Forest Essentials

~

PART IV
PEACE

Beauty comes with its own set of concomitant worries—a new breakout, the first wrinkle, the shock of white hair. Most often we fear losing youth as we feel it is synonymous with beauty. Conversely, worrying makes us look older. It gives us frown lines, a tight mouth and a lack of joie de vivre, and all of this can age even a teenager. When we're relaxed we radiate a sense of comfort and lightness, which makes us effortlessly attractive. But when we hold on to anger, grudges and disappointments, it shrouds our aura like a dark cloud.

Peace is the most vital element of beauty, but it's also the most elusive.

Our mind jumps from one thought to another faster than the speed of light. It has the tendency to always find something to fret about: when we don't have money, we yearn for luxury. When we have luxury, we want simplicity. When we are in a relationship, we miss being on our own. And when we have beauty, we worry about losing it. Our mind keeps us going around in circles—the more we follow its lead, the more it ties us up in knots.

When we're unhappy, abused or agitated over a period of time, beauty goes first. We become so entangled in our inner darkness that it envelops every cell, shutting off the light that gives us our inner glow. In those times, more than others, it is essential to hold on to hope and develop a practice where the mind does not completely take over the body.

Meditation is one tool that helps us control our mind so that we don't drown in a whirlpool of worry. Most people think they cannot meditate because they think too much. They may be right. But we can always begin by breathing deeply and focusing on each and every breath for five minutes. This disconnects us from stress. We can also look for an activity that engrosses us to an extent that we don't think of anything else. It could be pottery, painting or cooking— anything that is so absorbing that it makes us feel renewed. This too is meditation.

Or, at the very least, we must distance ourselves from our mind, observing our chain of thought like water flowing down a riverbed. Eventually, under the tutelage of a teacher, we can develop a meditation practice. Just like our bodies get used to exercise with regular practice, meditation helps control the mind when done with devotion and discipline.

Spiritual (not religious) practices give us an ethereal, otherworldly glow. We can eat all the superfoods or invest in the most expensive treatments, but they all fall flat when compared to the effects of a yogic lifestyle. When I say yogic I don't mean the practice of asanas, but activities that calm the mind and bring down inflammation. It could be prayer, pranayama, affirmations, healing practices or meditation.

I've dedicated a whole section to peace because without this element, beauty lacks resilience. If we're not inherently peaceful, anything can shatter our sense of well-being. Just like the sun scorches moisture off a freshly bloomed petal, constant agitation burns us from within, eliminating radiance by increasing inflammation. This is an often-ignored aspect, especially in today's world where we constantly look for instant gratification. When we take the time to centre and calm ourselves, it offers so many benefits that great skin will be insignificant, like husk on a grain of rice. Beauty will then be just a byproduct of happiness, stability and confidence, all of which come from a place of peace.

In this part I have selected aromatic spices and herbs that are known to relax the nervous system. However, these ingredients alone cannot make you peaceful because serenity is a choice, one that requires effort because it doesn't come easily.

31

SAFFRON (KESAR)

A few years ago I tried naturopathy for my endometriosis. Among the various herbs I was prescribed was saffron. I would add a few strands of it in a cup of tea and drink it every day. While this spice is supposed to be quite heating, I found it beneficial even in the peak of summer. Maybe it was my infatuation with this exotic spice or the placebo effect but I truly felt that it helped control my period pain and made my skin look calmer.

I always keep a jar of organic, A-grade saffron in my kitchen cabinet. I sometimes add it to tea, but after one friend told me that it closes pores I added a few strands to my rose water mist too. Only the stigma of the saffron flower is used, so about 150 flowers produce just 1 g of this spice. Even though it's prized for its colour and flavour, saffron offers much more than just cosmetic benefits.

Science

This spice contains minerals such as iron, manganese, zinc and selenium along with vitamins A and C, folic acid and carotenoids. I doubt if we get adequate amounts of vitamins and minerals from the minuscule amounts of saffron we consume. But its real health benefits lie in some of its volatile oils, namely safranal, and a carotenoid called a-crocin, which is responsible for its beautiful sunset colour.

The antioxidant capability of saffron is believed to reduce oxidative stress on the brain, changing the levels of mood-elevating neurotransmitters such as dopamine and serotonin. Another system of belief is that saffron is a mood-elevator because of its benefits on the gut—it strengthens the stomach, reduces acidity and improves digestion. Crocin and crocetin present in saffron have also been found to be good for the colon. In fact, they help reduce inflammation in ulcerative colitis. Our gut is also known as our second brain because the good bacteria can create mood-elevating neurotransmitters. The gut–brain axis is a bidirectional connection between the emotional centres of the brain and intestinal activity. Therefore, a healthy gut equals a healthy mind.

Saffron also has a healing effect on the liver—it protects it from oxidative stress, heals old damage and also reverses factors that can cause toxicity. We know by now that a well-functioning liver leads to clear skin. In addition, saffron has an anti-hyperglycaemic effect, which means that it helps reduce blood sugar levels.

There is strong evidence to suggest that taking 30 mg saffron capsules for a period of one to six months reduces the symptoms of depressive disorders. The effect was compared to drugs including fluoxetine[1] and imipramine.[2] Another study[3] conducted by Dr M. Agha-Hosseini and colleagues at the Tehran University of Medical Sciences found that supplementation with 15 mg saffron twice daily for two menstrual cycles halved the symptoms of premenstrual syndrome (PMS) in three-quarters of the participants. The aroma of the spice was also found to help in mildly reducing anxiety levels (about 10 per cent).[4] The antioxidant and anti-inflammatory effects of its constituents (safranal, crocin, crocetin) help in dealing with various nervous disorders including Alzheimer's and Parkinson's.[5] However, consult a naturopathic doctor before using it for a long term and at high doses.

It must be kept in mind that no one herb is responsible for bestowing a sense of peace. Feeling peaceful is an internal process and can be achieved with a mix of a healthy diet, exercise, positive relationships and fulfilling work. But more than that it's a result of your actions and the choices you make.

Tradition

Saffron is known as *kumkuma* in Ayurveda. It is the base for *kumkumadi tailam*—an important skin preparation in Ayurveda that brightens and tones the complexion. In the original kumkumadi preparation, all the sixteen herbs are supposed to represent the sixteen *kalas* (or phases) of the moon. The plucking of each herb is done on the kala that it is related to—saffron, of course, stands for the full moon.

There are many varieties of saffron. The Kashmiri type, which has a fragrance similar to the lotus, is considered to be the most superior. The Iranian or Turkish variant smells like honey and comes a close second. There is also a third type called Bahalik, from Afghanistan, that smells like *kewra* (pandanus flower).

Saffron is a purely sattvic spice that balances and calms the mind. It balances all the three doshas and falls in the varnya of complexion-enhancing herbs in Ayurveda. Its pungent and heating properties ensure that it penetrates deep into the tissue to deliver benefits. Even in Ayurveda, it is said to alleviate symptoms of depression and develop feelings of love and compassion in the heart.

Application

In the Indian tradition, it is used in diseases of the central nervous system, while Chinese medicine considers it to be a natural antidepressant. This just goes to prove one thing—traditional knowledge has always understood what modern science is yet to discover.

A lot of people say that this spice is very heating, however, we can enjoy 3–4 strands of saffron during winter and 2–3 strands in summer daily. The best vehicle or anupana to deliver the benefits of saffron is milk. Most herbs are best taken with fat because this helps to absorb the nutrients at a cellular level. Drinking turmeric water or saffron water will just wash it right out of your body—a complete waste of precious herbs, if you ask me. If you don't want to drink dairy then consume it with nut milk. But I believe that if you're not lactose-intolerant or do not suffer from inflammatory diseases, a small cup of good quality farm-fresh dairy milk may not be harmful. Milk has tryptophan, an essential amino acid that helps you sleep better. Therefore, this combination actually doubles the therapeutic effect of this calming spice.

Saffron helps reduce melanin formation and clarifies the complexion whether you eat or apply it. It can be mixed with a bit of sandalwood powder and applied on the face as a pack to brighten the complexion. You can also soak a few strands in 2 teaspoons of full-fat milk and leave on your face for 30 minutes. Then grind 5 almonds and apply to the skin for another 10 minutes. Dab with milk and scrub off gently. Finally wash off with milk and then water. Do keep in mind that you cannot use physical exfoliants like a scrub if you are using acid toners or peel pads.

Saffron induces sweating, so you can apply it as a body mask, which can have the same effect as taking a steam. Mix a fistful each of chickpea flour (besan) and boiled urad dal, and add a cup of saffron-infused milk. Apply all over the body and rub off when semi-dry. You can also infuse 4–5 threads of saffron in a cup (around 50 ml) of coconut oil with 1 teaspoon of sandalwood powder and a pinch of manjishtha powder. Keep this under the sun for 10–15 days. Store it in a dark amber glass bottle and use as a body oil.

Saffron improves focus and concentration. Just take a couple of threads and let them soak in a couple of drops of rose water. Then crush the threads with a spoon and apply the mixture in your eyes (like a kajal) before sleeping to soothe and rejuvenate them overnight. You may think that this will cause your skin to burn, but it has quite the opposite effect—you'll find it extremely cooling and clarifying.

Kashmiri Saffron Scrub

2 teaspoons coconut oil or almond oil or olive oil
A few strands of saffron
1 teaspoon castor sugar

- Mix all the ingredients together and make a paste.
- Gently scrub your face for 5 minutes.
- Wash it off with warm water.
- This scrub will instantly make your face glow and, over time, help reduce pigmentation.
- Use this scrub only if you are not using acids toners or peels pads.

32

HOLY BASIL (TULSI)

I first learnt about the amazing adaptogenic qualities of this pious herb when I met Professor Marc Cohen at the opening of Vana, one of India's leading wellness centres. Professor Cohen is one of Australia's leading experts in integrative and holistic medicine. Over cups of tea he explained why tulsi is as beneficial as green tea. Its lack of international recognition is only because it isn't marketed properly. He also told me that he grows tulsi plants in his house in Australia. He infuses handfuls of the leaves in water and carries a bottle to work to drink during the day.

For me the biggest benefit of tulsi tea is that it's not dehydrating. You can drink many cups of this tea and still feel hydrated and refreshed. I use tulsi like most people use caffeine—to feel awake. It's one of those rare herbs that makes you feel alert and relaxed at the same time. I always have a huge mug of tulsi tea next to me as I work. It makes me think better and be at peace. In fact, whenever I feel anxious, I slowly sip a cup and it makes me feel balanced again.

Science

Like any leafy herb, tulsi is also packed with vitamins A, C and K, along with various minerals such as calcium, manganese, magnesium, iron and zinc. However, the real strength of tulsi lies in its phytonutrients and volatile essential oils. It is probably the most researched herb for its radioprotective powers. A study found that its flavonoids protected mice from radiation-induced sickness and their tissues from tumours.[1] Even other phytochemicals such as eugenol, rosmarinic acid, apigenin and carnosic acid prevent radiation-induced DNA damage.

Tulsi increases the levels of antioxidants such as glutathione and enhances the effects of antioxidant enzymes such as superoxide dismutase,[2] which help protect the cells and tissues by mopping up damaging toxins. Therefore, this herb helps detoxify the body and fight against inflammation. While it protects the body against DNA damage by toxic compounds (pesticides, parabens, sulphates), it also helps the body get rid of these toxins by improving liver function. In addition, this wonderful herb guards us against heavy metals such as lead and arsenic, making it a complete shield for the body.

These days we live a sedentary lifestyle, with poor diets and increased mental pressures, because of which we have metabolic stress. This makes us prone to several chronic lifestyle diseases such as hypertension, obesity, diabetes, etc. Tulsi reduces blood glucose, balances the lipid profile, prevents weight gain and protects organs such as our liver, kidneys and pancreas. It also works as an antibacterial, antifungal and antiviral agent, thereby boosting the body's natural immunity. For these reasons tulsi is not just an option but also an absolute essential to fight the effects of pollution that comes from air, food, water, cosmetics and even internal stress.

Dr Cohen likes to refer to tulsi as 'liquid yoga' because it really does make the mind calmer and provides clarity of thought. I've experienced it personally, and perhaps can feel it more because I stay away from stimulants such as caffeine. The big difference between a caffeinated drink and tulsi is that firstly, this herb is not habit-forming. Secondly, while caffeine is stimulating, tulsi is more grounding and awakening. So while you will feel alert, it will come with a sense of calmness and not jitters. For this reason and many more, tulsi will always be a part of my kitchen cabinet.

Tradition

The word tulsi means 'the incomparable one'. This purely sattvic herb has been revered for thousands of years and is considered the most sacred plant in India. Every home has a tulsi plant that is supposed to be worshipped each morning. More often than not there is a scientific reason behind most traditions. Tulsi's detoxifying capabilities apply not just to the human body but also to the environment. So you could say that this plant is sort of a natural air purifier for the house.

There's a belief that one should not chew its leaves because tulsi is considered to be Lord Vishnu's wife. Here too, there is a bit of science behind what looks like superstition. Tulsi leaves have a high mercury content and can therefore damage the tooth enamel if chewed regularly. You can swallow the leaf or drink the tea but not chew the leaves on a regular basis.

As far as taste is concerned, tulsi is pungent (heating and penetrating) and bitter (cooling and detoxifying). So you can see from an Ayurvedic perspective that it has the capability to go deep into the tissues and detoxify them. While it's reasonably safe for everyone to use, in excess, tulsi's heating quality can increase pitta dosha (characterized by redness in the skin). For pitta types, it's best to take tulsi tea with a cooling herb like mint.

Application

There are different types of tulsi leaves. The tulsi plant in our homes is holy basil. Sweet basil is *vana tulsi*, while the purple-tinged plant is the *Krishna tulsi*. The genus is the same but the species are different. The prabhava or special power of holy basil is that it is antimicrobial. Tulsi has an ingredient called ursolic acid, which revives and repairs damaged cells. You can add a bit to your face mask, toss it in salads or drink it as a tea for its antioxidant, anti-inflammatory benefits. When you apply tulsi make sure you mix it with curd or multani mitti to cool it down. If you're tired or burnt out after office, swallow one crushed black peppercorn with 4–5 tulsi leaves to revive yourself. In fact, tulsi seeds are also very good for deworming and can be whisked in salads and yoghurt.

Sweet basil increases sweating and thus helps reduce high body temperature. One thing to keep in mind is to never boil the leaves with water. Make an infusion by pouring hot water over the leaves. Using a tulsi teabag is fine, but boiling reduces its active ingredients. Sweet basil is also an excellent appetizer. If you drink 1 teaspoon of the juice half an hour before your meals you'll find that your appetite increases. Krishna tulsi is even more powerful in potency as compared to the other two varieties. People don't consume it generally because it has a very sharp taste. But it is an excellent houseplant as it protects against pollution and wards off mosquitoes.

Did you know?

Tulsi is a great pain-relieving agent. You'll get relief from mild pain by consuming 2–3 leaves of crushed tulsi leaves with 1 teaspoon of ginger juice.

33

GOTU KOLA

This wonderful herb is part of most Ayurvedic skincare formulations. I use a toner and face mask containing gotu kola. So it is safe to assume that it's quite an inherent part of my life. I also drink a tea made with tulsi and gotu kola. Together these two herbs make me feel calm, grounded and focussed. Often this herb gets confused with brahmi. Even in some traditional texts both herbs are called 'brahmi'. However, they are different. Gotu kola has round, scalloped leaves with the stem joining the centre of the leaf. Brahmi, on the other hand, has oblong leaves and tiny white flowers. Both of them work on the mind but are still very different from each other.

I love products made with gotu kola, especially face masks. They stimulate the skin and make it glow. However, unlike other stimulatory ingredients, this herb does not make the skin look red and inflamed, unless of course if you're allergic to it—I, for one, am not. A lot of people say that gotu kola helps develop the crown chakra (located right at the top of your head). But I feel that no one herb is an answer to spiritual enlightenment. However, drinking gotu kola tea does make me feel calmer and centred. From a beauty perspective, when you are relaxed, your skin and hair naturally behave themselves. You look more beautiful because you're at peace with yourself.

Science

While gotu kola contains several vitamins and minerals, like any nutraceutical, its real strength lies in its phytochemical composition. Its active ingredients are saponins called centellosides (asiatic acid, madecassic acid and asiaticosides). In animal studies these compounds have been found to speed up wound healing and increase tensile strength in both cuts and burns via topical application.[1] Gotu kola is known to increase blood circulation, and is therefore used to reduce swelling on the legs due to lack of movement. The herb boosts collagen and encourages hyaluronic acid synthesis.[2] Because of these reasons it is a popular ingredient in beauty products.

Animal studies[3] have also shown that this herb acts as a sedative. In one human study[4] it was found that people who took it were less startled by a new noise than those who took a placebo. Since this could be one way to find out if a person is anxious, some presume gotu kola may help reduce symptoms of anxiety. Another study published in *Evidence-Based Complementary and Alternative Medicine*[5] found that gotu kola extract is effective in improving cognitive function after a stroke. Animal studies[6] have also shown this herb's potential as an antidepressant. However, while it is safe to take it for a few months at a time or to apply it on the skin, supplements must be taken after consulting an Ayurvedic doctor as they may interfere with certain medications.

Tradition

The great thing about nature is that a plant usually mimics the appearance of the organ it benefits the most. For instance, kidney beans are excellent for the kidneys and walnuts boost brainpower. Gotu kola is also called *saraswati* because it enhances the memory. It is shaped like the brain, and was traditionally considered to be the ultimate tonic to enhance mental faculties. It was used to treat brain disorders, soothe frayed nerves and also heal skin diseases. It is one of the four *medhya rasayanas* or brain rejuvenators, the others being brahmi, *shankha pushpi* and *jyotishmati*.

Gotu kola is sattvic (balancing) in nature and has a cooling effect on the mind and body. When applied on the skin it heals infections and acne. Legend has it that many Indian yogis and Chinese herbalists who consumed this herb regularly went on to live for more than a hundred years. It refreshes brain health and memory, protects the nervous system, strengthens capillaries, improves circulation, builds immunity and increases physical energy.

Note: A lot of brahmi supplements are actually gotu kola. You just have to look at the list of ingredients for the scientific name. Gotu kola is *Centella asiatica* while brahmi is *Bacopa monnieri.*

Application

The best way to consume this herb is to extract its juice from the leaf (about 10–20 ml) and drink it on an empty stomach in the morning. This helps people with anxiety. You can also eat less than 1 teaspoon of gotu kola powder with honey or mishri to calm down burning sensations. If you are a kapha person (prone to cold, cough or weight gain), take it with a pinch of warming spice or herb like 2–3 tulsi leaves.

You can mix it with a little aloe vera pulp and apply on inflamed spots as it aids wound healing. If you have a pimple (not hormonal or cystic), you can apply it and leave it on for the day. People with liver disorders, high blood pressure and pregnant women should only consume it under the supervision of a medical doctor.

Burmi Saag

2 cups fresh gotu kola leaves
½ teaspoon cumin seeds
4–5 garlic pods, chopped
1–2 green chillies
Mustard oil

- Toss the gotu kola leaves, cumin seeds, garlic and green chillies in mustard oil until the leaves have wilted.
- Eat it as a side dish.

34

WHITE PUMPKIN (PETHA)

Come summer and your palate changes. From enjoying dark leafy vegetables cooked in pungent mustard oil, you yearn for something cool and refreshing. Over the years I have learnt to relish tasteless summer vegetables. A light bottle gourd (*ghia*) curry is a real treat for me. But even those who turn up their noses at these veggies will still appreciate a sweet and sour pumpkin preparation.

I always prefer to buy the white variety (also called ash gourd) and cook it with the Bengali panchphoran, turmeric, salt, a bit of sugar and whole red chillies. I eat this with amaranth rotis. This meal makes me feel clean and light even on the hottest summer day.

Pumpkin has always been considered the healthiest of vegetables, especially its orange or yellow variety that comes with a high vitamin A content. However, from a spiritual perspective, the white pumpkin is considered the most superior of all climbing vegetables.

Science

Don't let the white colour fool you. Despite the bland shade, it's still a powerhouse of nutrients including vitamins A, C, E and K. It also contains a mix of B vitamins, manganese, copper and zinc. Ash gourd is a great source of lutein (also present in marigold) that is extremely beneficial for the eyes. Animal studies have shown that white pumpkin inhibits the development of ulcers,[1] protects the kidneys[2] and even has antidepressant properties.[3] This vegetable is packed with fibre and contains zero cholesterol and is hence extremely useful in cardiovascular diseases.

White pumpkin also contains L-tryptophan, an essential amino acid that the body cannot produce on its own. Put simply, tryptophan raises the serotonin levels in the body. Low levels of serotonin are considered a major cause of depression. However, I must say that no one vegetable can work as the cure for your blues. These are just handy tools that go well with a healthy lifestyle.

Tradition

In the *Ashtanga Samgraha*, the great sage Vagbhata calls white pumpkin the best out of all creepers. It's sweet in taste, which means that it's nourishing for the tissues, and has a cooling effect. Its special power or prabhava is that it sharpens the intellect. White pumpkin is also a *medhya dravya* (food for the brain) that improves your memory. It cools you down and makes you more alert and intelligent. It's useful in urinary tract infections, improves digestion and increases strength and immunity. It destroys excess pitta and vata. However, if you are prone to weight gain, you must take it for short periods only.

Traditionally it was used for diseases of the mind and nerves. The juice of white pumpkin is highly recommended to keep yourself calm and balanced. Even in Unani medicine it is considered a brain tonic. Since it is also appreciated for its blood-clotting properties, it is given along with amla or lime juice to control profuse bleeding. White pumpkin juice is also prescribed to calm down excessive aggression. In my experience, most beauty is destroyed by anger and aggression, whether you face it from others or burn yourself with negativity from within.

Application

If you're consuming the pulp, eat 10–20 g as a therapeutic dose. If you have a burning sensation, you can consume a full glass of juice. White pumpkin is good for rosacea because of its cooling nature. If you're taking the seeds, you can eat about 20–25 every day, or a heaped teaspoon of their powder. You can also mix the seeds in a laddu or muesli.

Every food has a thermogenic effect associated with it. Every time we eat food, various reactions take place in our body to utilize the nutrients. Your body usually requires 2–3 hours to absorb vitamins, but with white pumpkin you can get them in as little as 30 minutes. This is because it is utilized very smoothly by the body. It doesn't increase sugar levels and is instantly revitalizing because the body has to do very little work to digest it. It is great for women with PCOS or acne.

You can add it to soups, curries, sides or drink its juice. White pumpkin is extremely alkaline and really helps soothe the mind and clarify the skin.

White Pumpkin Poriyal

1 large cup white pumpkin
1 medium onion, chopped
1 green chilli, chopped
½ teaspoon mustard seeds
½ teaspoon cumin seeds
½ teaspoon turmeric powder
2 sprigs of curry leaves
¾ cup grated coconut
1–1½ tablespoons coconut oil
Salt to taste

- Chop the pumpkin and keep it aside with the chopped onions and green chilli.
- In a pan, heat the coconut oil. Then add the mustard seeds. When they pop, add the cumin seeds. When the cumin seeds start to sizzle in the hot oil, add the onion. Fry the onion till transparent.
- Add the curry leaves and green chilli. Fry for some seconds.
- Now add the pumpkin.
- Add the turmeric powder and sauté for a minute.

- Cover the pan and let the pumpkin cook in its own juice. Do not add water as the vegetable has enough water in it. Cook for 7–8 minutes till it is almost done. Then add the grated coconut.
- Mix the coconut well with the vegetable. Add salt and cook covered for a couple of minutes.
- Serve as a side dish or with dal and rice or sambar and rice.

White Pumpkin South Indian Kadhi

⅓ cup arhar dal (wash in water at least 3–4 times)
2 tablespoons black peppers
1 tablespoon whole cumin seeds
½ cup white pumpkin, cut into ½-inch cubes
4 green chillies, slit lengthwise
⅓ cup grated coconut
6 curry leaves
2 cups fresh curd
½ teaspoon cold-pressed cooking oil
½ teaspoon turmeric powder
2 tablespoons virgin coconut oil
A pinch of turmeric powder
A pinch of fenugreek seeds
2 teaspoons salt

- Soak the dal, pepper, green chillies and cumin seeds together in 1 cup water for 10 minutes. Grind all the soaked ingredients along with the grated coconut and the retained water into a grainy paste.

- Boil the white pumpkin in ½ cup water after adding the turmeric powder for 3–4 minutes without covering the pan. Turn off the gas and retain the water.
- In a saucepan, heat the cooking oil. Add the ground paste and give it a stir for a couple of minutes. Pour in the curd slowly and keep stirring it on medium heat for about 5–6 minutes. It is important to keep stirring continuously to avoid curdling of the curd. When the mixture comes to a boil, lower the heat and add the white pumpkin along with its water plus 4 extra cups of water. Now add the salt. Stir on low heat for a couple of minutes and turn off the gas.
- Heat 2 tablespoons of coconut oil. Then add the curry leaves along with the fenugreek seeds and turmeric. When it splutters, add to the kadhi and immediately close the lid. This will help keep the flavours intact.

35

BHRINGRAJ

For the last couple of years I've been regularly oiling my hair. I like to leave the hair oil on for a couple of hours at least before I shampoo it off. Even when I don't have time, I leave it on for 20–30 minutes. I've tried several types of oils but the one I regularly use is bhringraj. It has made my hair much thicker, boosted its growth and slowed down the greying process.

My mother is severely allergic to hair colour. The coin-sized welts on her neck and forehead every time she applies chemical colour is proof of how toxic it really is. She usually applies henna and indigo one after the other (for 45 minutes each) to get a naturally dark hair colour. But if she gets even a touch up with chemical colour, her forehead starts burning immediately. So I try to stick to natural remedies to keep my hair looking as lush as possible. I find that when I use a good quality bhringraj oil, I don't even need a conditioner. But more than anything else this miraculous oil has greatly improved the quality of my scalp.

I used to wash my hair every alternate day with medicated shampoo because my scalp would get oily and flaky. But ever since I started using this oil, I only wash my hair twice a week. My scalp is healthy, non-flaky and barely gets oily. Unfortunately, most hairdressers and dermatologists strongly advise against oiling the hair. But I believe in traditional knowledge and would choose oil over a commercial product for scalp health. Bhringraj is backed by science too and there are studies to prove that it not only improves hair quality but also our overall well-being.

Science

I believe that traditional medicine has always known what modern science is proving today. It's no different with bhringraj. In our Ayurvedic texts it is recommended for baldness and greying. For hair growth, there's now proof that it could be as powerful as minoxidil—a popular formulation to stimulate hair growth. In a study on rodents published in *BioMed Research International*,[1] it was found that a petroleum extract with 2–5 per cent *Eclipta alba* (bhringraj) was more effective than 2 per cent minoxidil, which is the standard treatment for hair loss.

There are also animal studies to prove that bhringraj protects the liver. Not only does it restore liver function and heal lesions, but it has also shown some promise in regenerating liver cells. We also have research to prove that it has anti-diabetic,[2] anti-inflammatory and antioxidant benefits[3] because it has a huge range of phytonutrients. It contains triterpenoids (known for their anti-tumour, chemo-protective benefits, among many others), flavonoids (anti-allergic, antimicrobial, anti-inflammatory and antioxidant

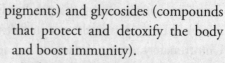

pigments) and glycosides (compounds that protect and detoxify the body and boost immunity).

Bhringraj is known for its ability to fight infections and parasites, which is why it was used to fight mosquito-borne infections such as malaria. It also boosts the immune system, making it an effective cure for skin diseases such as eczema. The benefits of this wonderful herb also go deep within the brain and nervous system. It's known to work as a sedative, muscle relaxant, memory booster and nerve strengthener. If hair fall and skin problems are caused by stress, then the relaxing quality of this herb will help control these problems.

Tradition

Traditionally this herb has been used not just in Ayurveda but also in Unani and Siddha medicine. Its main tastes are bitter (detoxifying and cooling) and pungent (warming and penetrating), therefore these opposites work to balance all the three doshas. It is also called false daisy (for its small flowers) and *kesharaj* as it has innumerable benefits for the hair.

Bhringraj falls under the category of rasayanas or rejuvenators. It is considered to be the ultimate anti-ager because it works on the skin, hair and also the internal tissues.

It helps purify the blood and break down ama (toxic waste) inside the body. It destroys harmful microbes and parasites, improves respiratory ailments such as asthma, helps with anaemic conditions and heals the liver too.

Application

The bhringraj oil I use is slowly simmered over twenty-one days with many Ayurvedic herbs. When applied, the oil feels cool on the head and has a calming effect on the mind. Among all the Ayurvedic preparations this is my absolute favourite for its undeniable benefits for the hair. One thing to keep in mind is that traditionally hair oil was always applied on a clean scalp, after washing the hair. Today people apply it on a dirty scalp. Perhaps that's why many experts say that it increases infection because dirt is the breeding ground for germs. If you want the full therapeutic benefits of hair oil, it is better to apply it on a relatively clean scalp. Think about it—would you apply cream on an unwashed face?

Many don't know that bhringraj powder takes care of urticaria as well, and helps even out the skin tone. If you have a scar, you can apply the bhringraj powder as a mask. Mix 1 teaspoon of the powder in fresh aloe vera juice and rose water and apply it on the spot. Let it semi-dry and then wash it off. Use it regularly for best effects. Bhringraj is so cooling and detoxifying that in earlier days it was also considered an antidote to snake venom. If you find fresh leaves you can eat 4–5 each morning to detoxify the body.

Bhringraj Hair Mask

1 cup dry bhringraj
2 tablespoons amla powder
2 tablespoons *reetha* powder
2 tablespoons shikakai powder
2 eggs

- Grind the dry bhringraj and mix it with the amla, reetha and shikakai powders.
- Mix this with the two eggs and apply on the hair. Leave it on for about an hour and then wash off with a gentle shampoo.
- Not only will this strengthen the hair but also give it lustre and shine.

36

JATAMANSI

The fragrance of this herb has something otherworldly about it. Just like sandalwood, *jatamansi* has a strong scent. It reminds you of incense but with a layer of mould on it. That's how it smells in its completely natural form, but you know that the right perfumer can extract the most fragrant oil out of this rare, precious herb. So rare that it's now endangered.

Jatamansi is prized because of its roots that look like a sage's dreadlocks. The act of ripping out the entire plant just for the roots and unregulated grazing of animals have led to its endangered status. Because it has such a wide range of benefits—from fragrance to haircare and as a mental tonic—about 75–80 per cent of jatamansi reserves have been depleted. While there are some biodynamic farms abroad that are trying to preserve this plant, I believe that its natural Himalayan habitat is responsible for its unique properties.

As we work on peace within we must show the same regard for our surroundings. It is important to use natural resources mindfully so that plants can thrive in their natural habitat. It is only then that we will be able to preserve our most powerful, medicinal herbs instead of using genetically modified versions that are devoid of healing qualities.

I feel that such potent, precious herbs should stop being used for merely cosmetic benefits. There are many other plants that can retexturize the skin and enhance hair quality. And there are others that make wonderful additions to fragrance. Jatamansi has such a profound effect on the mind that it must be used for this purpose alone.

Science

Also called musk root or spikenard, jatamansi is one of Ayurveda's most effective nervine tonics. It is commonly used as a mild sedative to reduce irritability, stress and nervousness. The best part of this rhizome is that despite its potent effects it is extremely safe to use (except on pregnant women due to lack of clinical trials). The herb can also be prescribed for children to reduce aggression and enhance memory. Today many animal studies prove its efficacy in reducing anxiety,[1] alleviating stress[2] and improving memory and learning[3] because of its high antioxidant content, which also helps to reduce inflammation.

Tradition

This potent herb has been revered in both Ayurvedic and Unani systems of medicine for years. Because its main tastes are bitter (cooling and detoxifying), astringent (cooling and toning) and sweet (cooling and nourishing), it reduces excess heat in the body and also calms the mind. It is tridoshic, i.e., it works to balance all the three doshas and is used as a mild sedative, memory enhancer and to bring about a sense of peace.

Application

Jatamansi helps reduce PMS symptoms and regularize ovulation. To utilize its sedative qualities, you must boil it in buffalo's milk. Even if it can't completely help you sleep, it will keep your mood stabilized the next day.

> **Calming bedtime drink**
>
> Boil 1 teaspoon of jatamansi powder in a cup of buffalo milk with 2–3 pinches of cardamom and 4–5 strands of saffron. Strain and drink the milk before you sleep.

37

CAMPHOR (KAPUR)

The fragrance of camphor has been an integral part of my life. Growing up, my mother would mix camphor along with other herbs to make a hair oil that would stimulate growth and improve scalp health. Later, as I got deeper into yoga and spirituality, I learnt that burning camphor reduces negativity in any space. Now I burn it at home, taking inspiration from my yoga guru, Seema Sondhi, who always burnt it at her studio.

My best friend, who comes from a family of Sanskrit scholars, keeps sachets of camphor in her car because she spends a lot of time driving. I have no experience of eating edible camphor and neither would I recommend it. Just the fragrance and application of this ancient spice is enough to heal the skin and rejuvenate the mind.

Science

Camphor or *kapur* has been used for decades for its decongesting, pain-relieving abilities. Synthetic camphor is an active ingredient in Vicks which, on application, opens up the nasal passages and relieves headaches when rubbed into the temples. It boosts circulation by producing both warming and cooling sensations. Increased circulation brings more nutrients under the skin's surface, thereby improving its health. Therefore, it is also a popular ingredient in beauty products.

Camphor reduces the sensation of itchiness on the skin. The cooling tingle of this spice calms down inflammation. However, it must never be applied on open wounds. It also works very well as an antiseptic, antibacterial and antifungal agent, which makes it an effective cure for acne, fungal infection and even dandruff. It is also a mild anaesthetic and sedative. This is perhaps the reason why it was used to pacify nervous conditions such as anxiety and mania in the past.

Tradition

Camphor is revered because it is believed to destroy negative energy. Its fragrance works like an insect repellent. Therefore, the practice of burning camphor at home has practical applications too. The tingling scent opens up the senses and clarifies a dull mind. I find the smell both soothing and energizing. It helps relax me, while keeping me awake and alert at the same time. Even in Ayurveda it is used to pacify the nervous system and get better sleep. Just the act of burning camphor and surrounding yourself with its unique aroma helps uplift the mind and remove negativity.

Application

While small amounts of this resin are ingested for various purposes in Ayurveda, I would not recommend that you take it without consulting an Ayurvedic doctor. When applied externally it helps reduce swelling, inflammation and pain, because of which camphor-infused oil was used in massages for arthritics.

There are three types of camphor: *bhimseni* (also called Borneo or Malay camphor), *kapur tulsi* (Indian camphor) and *cheeni kapur* (Chinese camphor). The first is the most effective and the third the least. Kapur tulsi has properties of both camphor and tulsi in it. Grown in the Himalayas, people even make a tea out of it. If you want camphor oil or need it to purify the house, look for the bhimseni variety.

Camphor increases the diameter of blood vessels and induces sweating, because of which it is extremely good for menopausal women when added to a carrier oil. It has a very soothing effect on burning hands and feet. Drop a couple of camphor pellets in about 50 ml of coconut oil and keep under the sun for 10–15 days. Use it as a hair or body oil. A pinch of good quality camphor added to your toothpaste works to reduce bad breath too.

For acne-prone skin, add 1 teaspoon of powdered medicinal camphor or camphor BP (camphor water) to 200 ml of rose water and wipe your face clean with this several times a day to prevent oil build-up. You can also make a paste of 2 teaspoons fuller's earth, ½ teaspoon camphor powder, 1 teaspoon fresh neem leaf paste and rose water and use it as a mask for oily skin.

Some people can develop rashes, so it's important to do a patch test before using camphor. Even if you're allergic to its application, you can still use it in your surroundings to purify the air and clear negativity.

38

SANDALWOOD (CHANDAN)

Like everyone who has ever delved into spirituality, I too became interested in it during one of the most stressful times of my life. In the beginning I wore crystals, tried various types of meditations and found myself a healer. Over the years I have reached a place where I am more relaxed. I still continue to practise and teach yoga, and I'm still spiritual—not out of desperation any more but from a place of love. The crystals have gone, along with the amulets and superstitions. What remains are my asana practice, meditation and belief in the powers of sandalwood.

I used to wear sandalwood paste on my forehead during the months when I was especially distraught. Religion had nothing to do with it. The application of the paste between my brows gave me a sense of confidence and calmed my mind. According to my healer, sandalwood enhances and protects your aura. Who knows how that really works but at that point in the past, it felt comforting to me.

Unfortunately sandalwood is now extremely endangered because of merciless felling. Its oil is perhaps more expensive than gold. So I find it surprising how many inexpensive products claim to contain this precious essence. While one may be able to synthetically copy its fragrance, most skin benefits come only from real, pure sandalwood.

Science

This aromatic wood has such a warm, earthy fragrance that it's a favourite among perfumers around the world. Some of the most iconic fragrances contain sandalwood essence. And when mixed with musk and gourmand notes like vanilla and tonka bean, it smells sensual and decadent. Whether it's simulation or tranquillity, sandalwood seems to work on both extremes in equal measure.

In a study[1] done on terminally ill patients, it was found that sandalwood oil showed some promise in reducing anxiety levels. Another study[2] found that aromatherapy with the oil increased markers of alertness such as pulse rate, perspiration, etc. So immense is the effect of sandalwood fragrance that a 2014 German study[3] published in the *Journal of Investigative Dermatology* found that just the smell of it activated the olfactory receptors in the skin that in turn prompted cells to proliferate and migrate. Put simply, just the smell of sandalwood (and that too synthetic) was enough to trigger the wound-healing process.

Tradition

Sandalwood sticks are an integral part of any religious ceremony. After the puja is done, the fresh stick is dampened and the paste applied to the centre of your forehead—right between the brows. Some people apply it to open the third eye, others to calm the mind. If you apply the paste on your forehead, you will find that it helps cool down the mind and the entire body.

In Ayurveda, sandalwood is known to improve the quality of skin and reduce burning sensations. It gets rid of body odour, relieves fatigue, gives courage and helps control the mind better. Sandalwood is a varnya (complexion-enhancing) herb so it improves the skin. It is also known as *shrikhand* because of the paste's creamy texture and colour.

Application

Apply sandalwood paste on the forehead after a stressful day to calm the mind. You can even dab the paste between your brows before you meditate. However, if you are a kapha personality, you should avoid sandalwood *tikka* as it may be too cooling for you. If you want to shield yourself from negativity, apply a bit of sandalwood oil at the base of your throat before you leave the house. Red sandalwood is a good remedy to fade acne marks—just mix it with aloe vera and apply it as a spot treatment once a day. Wash it off when semi-dry.

Sandalwood has a very earthy, grounding fragrance. It sets the mood for meditation and also makes me more focused. Just lighting good quality, pure chandan incense sticks relieves tension and adds joyousness to an otherwise mundane task. It's the ultimate beauty tool, the most enriching fragrance, and has the power to cool the entire body with just a dot in the centre of the forehead.

The sandalwood purity test

There is a test recommended by Acharya Bhavprakash to identify true sandalwood: the taste of real sandalwood will be bitter, and when you rub it with water it will give a yellowish, and not pinkish, hue like shrikhand. Sandalwood is light, dry, bitter, sweet and cooling.

~

'Peace and love are the biggest anti-agers. By love I don't mean being in love necessarily. It's more about being a loving person. As we age our skin doesn't regenerate as quickly. So while you may be able to get away with a lot of things when you are eighteen, as you grow older, your thoughts begin to show on your face. Some people look beautiful, but hard. It's their emotional baggage that rises to the surface. When you are not at peace and unhappy with yourself you create an inner conflict. You bombard yourself with fear, rage and resentment—feelings that distort beauty. On the contrary, when you are peaceful and content, you are calm and able to handle calamities with ease and grace. So even if you're not typically pretty, you have an inner glow that's magnetic. And with this calmness you're sure that, despite what happens, there is divine grace and that flowers will never stop blooming in your life.'

—Vivek Sahni, founder, Kama Ayurveda

~

शान्तितुल्यं तपो नास्ति न सन्तोषात्परं सुखम् ।
न तृष्णायाः परो व्याधिर्नच धर्मो दयात्परः॥

Shanti tulyam tapo naasti
Na santoshaatparam sukham
Na trishnaayaaha paro vyaadhih
Na cha dharmo dayaatparah

There is no self-purifying process equal to attaining
peace of mind, and no bliss equal to being satisfied
with one's lot. There is no disease bigger than
excessive desire or craving for worldly things, and
no tenet or religion greater than kindness towards all
living beings.

—Chanakya, *Chanakya Niti*

ACKNOWLEDGEMENTS

This book would not have been possible without the generosity of my expert panel, contributors, founders of beauty brands and the team at Penguin Random House India.

My editor, Gurveen Chadha, who guided me at every step, and Meena Rajasekaran, who designed a beautiful cover, which I will love for years to come.

My experts: Lovneet Batra, who went through all the chapters and corrected mistakes; Dr Ipsita Chatterjee, who gave me unique information that one cannot find easily in a book; Chef Sandeep Biswas, for his application tips and recipes; Dr Naresh Perumbuduri, for giving me information over the terrible connection at Tehri Garhwal; and Suparna Trikha, for all the beautifying tips and recipes.

All the contributors: Anjali and her mother, Anju, of Hema's Kitchen; Dr Akanksha Kotibhaskar and Aditi Bali of Forest Essentials; Dr Jyotsna Makker; my mom, Veena Singh, and my nani, Shanti Devi; my yoga guru, Seema Sondhi; Sunalini Matthew; Swati Kapoor of SoulTree; Carol Singh of Antidote; Divya Dugar; Neena Chopra of Just Herbs,

Lavanya Krishnan of The Boxwalla; Anuska Ilijic; Shubhika Jain of RAS Luxury Oils; Munmun Ganeriwal; Anju Rupal of Abhati Suisse; Bee Ham of H Is For Love; Kangan Badhwar; and Zahara Nedou of Zahara Skincare. Anita Mathur, for the recipe and the opening shloka; Himanshu Rai, for the idea of shlokas and the peace mantra; Ami Unnikrishnan and Prachee Satija, for helping out with the research; and Dhruv Kapur, who suggested a small but essential tweak in the pillars of beauty.

The founders of India's wellness and beauty brands: Bharat Mitra of Organic India, who opened the doors of his farm and helped me select the right ingredients; Kavita Khosa of Purearth, who taught me so much about natural beauty; Mira Kulkarni of Forest Essentials, who doesn't usually give interviews but made a special exception for my book; and Vivek Sahni, who indulged me in many conversations and imparted excellent advice.

Finally, Dr Nigma Talib for believing in me and being the very first person to review my book. And, most of all, Masaba Gupta for giving me an open-hearted foreword on our changing definition of beauty.

NOTES

Introduction

1. A.H. Maslow, 'A Theory of Human Motivation', *Psychological Review* 50 (1943): 370–96.

PART I: VITALITY

Coconut

1. Frank M. Sacks et al., 'Dietary Fats and Cardiovascular Disease: A Presidential Advisory from the American Heart Association', *Circulation*, 15 June 2017.

Mustard Oil

1. Sundeep Mishra and S.C. Manchanda, 'Cooking Oils for Heart Health', *Journal of Preventive Cardiology* 1 (2012): 123–31.

Ashwagandha

1. Chandrasekhar K., Kapoor J. and Anishetty S., 'A Prospective, Randomized Double-Blind, Placebo-Controlled Study of

Safety and Efficacy of a High-Concentration Full-Spectrum Extract of *Ashwagandha* Root in Reducing Stress and Anxiety in Adults', *Indian Journal of Psychological Medicine* 34 (2012): 255–62, doi: 10.4103/0253-7176.106022.

2. Wankhede S. et al., 'Examining the Effect of *Withania Somnifera* Supplementation on Muscle Strength and Recovery: A Randomized Controlled Trial', *Journal of the International Society of Sports Nutrition*, 25 November 2015.

PART II: CLARITY

Neem

1. Sonia Arora and Jananiga Vanniyasingam, 'Identification of Mechanism of Action of Anti-HIV Properties of Compounds Present in Neem (*Azadirachta indica*) Extracts', *The FASEB Journal*, 1 April 2012.

Katuki

1. Bedi K.L., Zutshi U., Chopra C.L. and Amla V., '*Picrorhiza Kurroa*, an Ayurvedic Herb, May Potentiate Photochemotherapy in Vitiligo', *Journal of Ethnopharmacology* 27 (1989): 347–52.

Triphala

1. Gurjar S., Pal A., Kapur S., 'Triphala and Its Constituents Ameliorate Visceral Adiposity from a High-Fat Diet in Mice with Diet-Induced Obesity', *Alternative Therapies in Health and Medicine* 18 (2012): 38–45.

2. Kamali S.H. et al., 'Efficacy of "Itrifal Saghir", a Combination of Three Medicinal Plants in the Treatment of Obesity; A Randomized Controlled Trial', *Daru* (2012): 33.

3. Saravanan S., 'Hypolipidemic Effect of Triphala in Experimentally Induced Hypercholesteremic Rats,' *Yakugaku Zasshi* 127 (2007): 385–88.

4. Patel D.K., Kumar R., Laloo D. and Hemalatha S., 'Diabetes Mellitus: An Overview on Its Pharmacological Aspects and Reported Medicinal Plants Having Antidiabetic Activity', *Asian Pacific Journal of Tropical Biomedicine* 2 (2012): 411–20.

Ginger and Garlic

1. Danwilai K., Konmun J., Sripanidkulchai B., Subongkot S., 'Antioxidant Activity of Ginger Extract as a Daily Supplement in Cancer Patients Receiving Adjuvant Chemotherapy: A Pilot Study,' *Cancer Management and Research* 9 (2017): 11–18, doi:10.2147/CMAR.S124016.

2. Queen's University, 'Chemists Shed Light on Health Benefits of Garlic', *ScienceDaily*, 31 January 2009, mwww.sciencedaily. com/releases/2009/01/090130154901.htm.

Aloe Vera

1. Cho S. et al., 'Dietary Aloe Vera Supplementation Improves Facial Wrinkles and Elasticity and It Increases the Type I Procollagen Gene Expression in Human Skin in vivo.', *Annals of Dermatology* 21 (2009): 6–11, doi: 10.5021/ad.2009.21.1.6.

2. Surjushe A., Vasani R. and Saple D.G., 'Aloe Vera: A Short Review', *Indian Journal of Dermatology* 53 (2008): 163–66.

Turnips and Radishes

1. Lee S.W. et al., 'Effects of White Radish (*Raphanus sativus*) Enzyme Extract on Hepatotoxicity', *Toxicological Research* 28 (2012): 165–72. doi: 10.5487/TR.2012.28.3.165.

2. Banihani S.A., 'Radish (*Raphanus sativus*) and Diabetes', *Nutrients* 9 (2017): 1014, doi: 10.3390/nu9091014.
3. Jibran Khatri et al., 'It Is Rocket Science—Why Dietary Nitrate Is Hard to 'Beet'! Part I: Twists and Turns in the Realization of the Nitrate–Nitrite–NO Pathway', *British Journal of Clinical Pharmacology* 83 (2016): 129–39.

Giloi

1. Saha S. and Ghosh S., '*Tinospora cordifolia*: One Plant, Many Roles', *Ancient Science of Life* 31 (2012): 151–59, doi: 10.4103/0257-7941.107344.
2. Badar V.A. et al., 'Efficacy of *Tinospora cordifolia* in Allergic Rhinitis,' *Journal of Ethnopharmacology* 96 (2005): 445–49.

Wheatgrass

1. Satyavati Rana, Jaspreet Kaur Kamboj and Vandana Gandhi, 'Living Life the Natural Way—Wheatgrass and Health', *Functional Foods in Health and Disease* 1 (2011): 444–56.
2. Marawaha R.K., Bansal D., Kaur S. and Trehan A., 'Wheat Grass Juice Reduces Transfusion Requirement in Patients with Thalassemia Major: A Pilot Study'. *Indian Pediatrics* 41 (2004): 716–20.

PART III: RADIANCE

Moringa

1. Kushwaha S., Chawla P. and Kochhar A., 'Effect of Supplementation of Drumstick (*Moringa oleifera*) and Amaranth (*Amaranthus tricolor*) Leaves Powder on Antioxidant

Profile and Oxidative Status among Postmenopausal Women,' *Journal of Food Science and Technology* 51 (2014): 3464–69, doi: 10.1007/s13197-012-0859-9.

Indian Berries

1. Jyoti Sinha, Shalini Purwar, Kumar Satya Chuhan and Gyanendra Rai, 'Nutritional and Medicinal Potential of *Grewia subinaequalis DC. (syn. G. asiatica.)* (Phalsa)', *Journal of Medicinal Plants Research* 9 (2015): 594–612, doi: 10.5897/JMPR2015.5724.

2. Bernstein A.M., Roizen M.F. and Martinez L., 'Purified Palmitoleic Acid for the Reduction of High-Sensitivity C-Reactive Protein and Serum Lipids: A Double-Blinded, Randomized, Placebo-Controlled Study', *Journal of Clinical Lipidology* 8 (2014): 612–17, doi: 10.1016/j.jacl.2014.08.001.

3. R. Zadernowski et al., 'Composition of Phenolic Acids in Sea Buckthorn (*Hippophae rhamnoides L.*) Berries', *Journal of the American Oil Chemists' Society* 82 (2005): 175, doi: 10.1007/s11746-005-5169-1.

Indian Seeds

1. Asim Sarfraz et al., 'Study of Inhibitory Effect of Extract of Ajwain (*Trachyspermum ammi*) on Candida Albicans', *International Journal of Contemporary Medical Research* 3 (2016): 2851–52.

2. Shim S.H. et al., 'Rat Growth-Hormone Release Stimulators from Fenugreek Seeds', *Chemistry & Biodiversity* 5 (2008): 1753–61, doi: 10.1002/cbdv.200890164.

3. Fuller S. and Stephens J.M., 'Diosgenin, 4-Hydroxyisoleucine, and Fiber from Fenugreek: Mechanisms of Actions and

Potential Effects on Metabolic Syndrome', *Advances in Nutrition* 6 (2015): 189–97, doi: 10.3945/an.114.007807.

Marigold (Genda)

1. Kang C.H., Rhie S.J. and Kim Y.C., 'Antioxidant and Skin Anti-Aging Effects of Marigold Methanol Extract', *Toxicological Research* 34 (2018): 31–39, doi: 10.5487/ TR.2018.34.1.031.

Bitter Apricots

1. Keyou Li et al., 'Bitter Apricot Essential Oil Induces Apoptosis of Human HaCaT Keratinocytes', *International Immunopharmacology* 34 (2016): 189–98, doi: 10.1016/j. intimp.2016.02.019.

PART IV: PEACE

Saffron (Kesar)

1. Akhondzadeh Basti A. et al., 'Comparison of Petal of *Crocus sativus L.* and Fluoxetine in the Treatment of Depressed Outpatients: A Pilot Double-Blind Randomized Trial', *Progress in Neuro-Psychopharmacology & Biological Psychiatry* 31 (2007): 439–42.
2. Akhondzadeh S. et al., 'Comparison of *Crocus sativus L.* and Imipramine in the Treatment of Mild to Moderate Depression: A Pilot Double-Blind Randomized Trial', *BMC Complementary and Alternative Medicine* 4 (2004): 12, doi: 10.1186/1472-6882-4-12.
3. Agha-Hosseini M. et al., '*Crocus sativus L.* (Saffron) in the Treatment of Premenstrual Syndrome: A Double-Blind,

Randomized and Placebo-Controlled Trial,' *BJOG* 115 (2008): 515–19, doi: 10.1111/j.1471-0528.2007.01652.x.

4. Fukui H., Toyoshima K. and Komaki R., 'Psychological and Neuroendocrinological Effects of Odour of Saffron (*Crocus sativus*)', *Phytomedicine* 18 (2011): 726–30, doi: 10.1016/j.phymed.2010.11.013.

5. Khazdair M.R. et al., 'The Effects of *Crocus sativus* (Saffron) and Its Constituents on Nervous System: A Review,' *Avicenna Journal of Phytomedicine* 5 (2015): 376–91.

Holy Basil (Tulsi)

1. Baliga M.S., Rao S., Rai M.P. and D'souza P., 'Radio Protective Effects of the Ayurvedic Medicinal Plant *Ocimum sanctum Linn.* (Holy Basil): A Memoir', *Journal of Cancer Research and Therapeutics* 12 (2016): 20–27, doi: 10.4103/0973-1482.151422.

2. M.M. Cohen, 'Tulsi—*Ocimum sanctum*: A Herb for All Reasons', *Journal of Ayurveda and Integrative Medicine* 5 (2014): 251–59, doi: 10.4103/0975-9476.146554.

Gotu Kola

1. Bylka W., Znajdek-Awiżeń P., Studzińska-Sroka E. and Brzezińska M, '*Centella asiatica* in Cosmetology', *Advances in Dermatology and Allergology/Postępy Dermatologii I Alergologii* 30 (2013): 46–49, doi: 10.5114/pdia.2013.33378.

2. Ibid.

3. Somboonwong J., Kankaisre M., Tantisira B. and Tantisira M.H., 'Wound Healing Activities of Different Extracts of *Centella asiatica* in Incision and Burn Wound Models: An Experimental Animal Study', *BMC Complementary and Alternative Medicine* 12 (2012): 103, doi: 10.1186/1472-6882-12-103.

4. Bradwejn J., Zhou Y., Koszycki D. and Shlik J., 'A Double-Blind, Placebo-Controlled Study on the Effects of Gotu Kola (*Centella asiatica*) on Acoustic Startle Response in Healthy Subjects', *J Clin Psychopharmacol.* 20 (2000): 680–84.

5. Farhana K.M., Malueka R.G., Wibowo S. and Gofir A., 'Effectiveness of Gotu Kola Extract 750 mg and 1000 mg Compared with Folic Acid 3 mg in Improving Vascular Cognitive Impairment after Stroke', *Evidence-Based Complementary and Alternative Medicine* 2016 (2016): 2795915, doi: 10.1155/2016/2795915.

6. Chen Y. et al., 'Effects of Total Triterpenes of *Centella asiatica* on the Corticosterone Levels in Serum and Contents of Monoamine in Depression Rat Brain', *Zhong Yao Cai* 28 (2005): 492–26.

White Pumpkin (Petha)

1. Rachchh M.A. and Jain S.M., 'Gastroprotective Effect of *Benincasa hispida* Fruit Extract', *Indian Journal of Pharmacology* 40 (2008): 271–75, doi: 10.4103/0253-7613.45154.

2. Manoj S. Pagare, Leena Patil and Vilasrao J. Kadam, '*Benincasa hispida*: A Natural Medicine', *Research Journal of Pharmacy and Technology* 4 (2011): 1941–44.

3. Dhingra D. and Joshi P., 'Antidepressant-Like Activity of *Benincasa hispida* Fruits in Mice: Possible Involvement of Monoaminergic and GABAergic Systems', *Journal of Pharmacology & Pharmacotherapeutics* 3 (2012): 60–62, doi: 10.4103/0976-500X.92521.

Bhringraj

1. Begum S. et al., 'Comparative Hair Restorer Efficacy of Medicinal Herb on Nude (Foxn1nu) Mice', *BioMed*

Research International 2014 (2014): 319795, doi: 10.1155/2014/319795.

2. Ananthi J., Prakasam A. and Pugalendi K.V., 'Antihyperglycemic Activity of *Eclipta alba* Leaf on Alloxan-Induced Diabetic Rats', *Yale Journal of Biology and Medicine* 76 (2003): 97–102.

3. Rownak Jahan, Abdullah Al-Nahain, Snehali Majumder and Mohammed Rahmatullah, 'Ethnopharmacological Significance of *Eclipta alba* (L.) Hassk. (Asteraceae),' *International Scholarly Research Notices* 2014 (2014), doi: 10.1155/2014/385969.

Jatamansi

1. N. Deepak Venkataraman and P. Muralidharan, 'Evaluation of Anti-Anxiety Activity of *Nardostachys jatamansi* Rhizomes,' *International Journal of Green Pharmacy* 1 (2007): 26–29.

2. Nazmun Lyle et al., 'Stress Modulating Antioxidant Effect of *Nardostachys jatamansi*', *Indian Journal of Biochemistry & Biophysics* 46 (2009): 93–98.

3. Joshi H. and Parle M., '*Nardostachys jatamansi* Improves Learning and Memory in Mice', *Journal of Medicinal Food* (2006): 113–18.

Sandalwood (Chandan)

1. Kyle G., 'Evaluating the Effectiveness of Aromatherapy in Reducing Levels of Anxiety in Palliative Care Patients: Results of a Pilot Study', *Complementary Therapies in Clinical Practice* 12 (2006): 148–55.

2. Heuberger E., Hongratanaworakit T. and Buchbauer G., 'East Indian Sandalwood and alpha-Santalol Odor Increase Physiological and Self-Rated Arousal in Humans', *Planta Medica* 72 (2006): 792–800.

3. Busse D. et al., 'A Synthetic Sandalwood Odorant Induces Wound-Healing Processes in Human Keratinocytes via the Olfactory Receptor OR2AT4', *Journal of Investigative Dermatology* 134 (2014): 2823–32. doi: 10.1038/jid.2014.273.

BIBLIOGRAPHY

Bhaskar, Dr Bhaswati. *Everyday Ayurveda: Daily Habits That Can Change Your Life*. New Delhi: Random House India, 2015.

Ghai, C.M. *Health Rejuvenation and Longevity through Ayurveda*. New Delhi: Deep & Deep Publications, 2004.

Frawley, Dr David. *Ayurveda and the Mind: The Healing of Consciousness*. New Delhi: Motilal Banarsidass, 2005.

Frawley, Dr David and Dr Vasant Lad. *The Yoga of Herbs: An Ayurvedic Guide to Herbal Medicine*. Wisconsin, United States: Lotus Press, 2001.

Murthy, Srikantha K.R. *Astanga Samgraha of Vagbhata*. Varanasi: Chaukhamba Orientalia, 2012.

Sharma, R.K. and Bhagwan Dash. *Caraka Samhita* (Text with English Translation and Critical Exposition Based on Cakrapani Datta's *Ayurveda Dipika*). Varanasi: Chowkhamba Sanskrit Series Office, 2014.

LIST OF CONTRIBUTORS

PART I: VITALITY

Ghee

- Balancing medicated ghee recipe and Ayurvedic and application inputs by Dr Naresh Perumbuduri, senior Ayurvedic physician, Ananda in the Himalayas, Uttarakhand.
- Nutrition inputs by Lovneet Batra, founder, Arbhavya, Delhi.

Coconut

- Coconut and clay toothpaste recipe by Divya Dugar, film-maker, zero-waste expert and co-author of *Slumgirl Dreaming: Rubina's Journey to the Stars*.
- Mom's nourishing coconut oil recipe by Veena Singh.
- Amma's coconut chutney recipe by Hema Gupta, founder, Hema's South Indian.
- Coconut milk recipe by Carol Singh, founder, Antidote.
- Ayurvedic and application inputs by Dr Naresh Perumbuduri.
- Nutrition and application inputs by Lovneet Batra.

Mustard Oil

- Ayurvedic and application inputs by Dr Naresh Perumbuduri.
- Nutrition and application inputs by Lovneet Batra.
- Application inputs by Suparna Trikha, natural beauty expert and director, Suparna Herbs India Pvt. Ltd.

Sattu

- Ayurvedic inputs by Dr Jyotsna Makker, founder, Tanmatra Ayurveda, Gurugram.
- Nutrition and application inputs by Lovneet Batra.
- Application inputs by Chef Sandeep Biswas, wellness chef, India.

Millets

- Exfoliating body cleanser powder recipe by Dr Neena Chopra, director, beauty and technical, Just Herbs.
- Nani's warming bajra khichdi recipe by Shanti Devi.
- Express ragi breakfast drink, black rice and ragi puttu recipes by Sunalini Matthew, health and wellness journalist.
- Ragi idli recipe by Hema Gupta.
- Millet breakfast brownies recipe by Anuska Iljic, vinyasa and yin yoga teacher and garbologist.
- Application inputs by Chef Sandeep Biswas
- Nutrition and application inputs by Lovneet Batra and Munmun Ganeriwal, dietician, nutritionist and fitness consultant, Mumbai.

Rice

- Brown rice dosa recipe by Hema Gupta.

- Black rice glow bowl recipe by Sunalini Matthew.
- Ayurvedic and application inputs by Dr Naresh Perumbuduri.
- Nutrition and application inputs by Lovneet Batra.
- Application inputs by Chef Sandeep Biswas.

Raw Honey

- Oatmeal and honey face scrub recipe by Shubhika Jain, founder, RAS Luxury Oils.
- Ayurvedic and application inputs by Dr Naresh Perumbuduri.
- Nutrition and application inputs by Lovneet Batra.
- Application inputs by Chef Sandeep Biswas.

Jaggery (Gur)

- Ayurvedic inputs by Dr Naresh Perumbuduri.
- Nutrition inputs by Lovneet Batra.
- Application inputs by Chef Sandeep Biswas.
- Winter jaggery snack recipe and application inputs by Munmun Ganeriwal.

Ashwagandha

- Ayurvedic and application inputs by Dr Naresh Perumbuduri.
- Nutrition and application inputs by Lovneet Batra.
- Application inputs by Chef Sandeep Biswas.

Munakka

- Ayurvedic inputs by Dr Naresh Perumbuduri.
- Nutrition and application inputs by Lovneet Batra.
- Application inputs by Chef Sandeep Biswas.

Tragacanth Gum (Gond)

- Ayurvedic inputs by Dr Naresh Perumbuduri.
- Nutrition and application inputs by Lovneet Batra.
- Gluten-free gond laddu and summer gond cooler recipes by Chef Sandeep Biswas.

PART II: CLARITY

Neem

- Gut-cleansing neem begun recipe by Dr Ipsita Chatterjee.
- Skin-clearing neem steam recipe by Anju Rupal.
- Purifying neem tea recipe by Dr Akanksha Kotibhaskar, Ayurveda consultant, Forest Essentials.
- Ayurvedic and application inputs by Dr Ipsita Chatterjee.
- Nutrition inputs by Lovneet Batra.

Manjishtha

- Tone-clearing manjishtha lep recipe by Dr Akanksha Kotibhaskar.
- Ayurvedic and application inputs by Dr Ipsita Chatterjee.
- Nutrition inputs by Lovneet Batra.

Katuki

- Ayurvedic and application inputs by Dr Naresh Perumbuduri.
- Nutrition inputs by Lovneet Batra.

Triphala

- Triphala recipe by Chef Sandeep Biswas.
- Ayurvedic and application inputs by Dr Naresh Perumbuduri.

- Nutrition inputs by Lovneet Batra.

Turmeric (Haldi)

- White turmeric brightening mask recipe by Bee Ham, founder, H Is For Love.
- Kasturi manjal glow mask recipe by Dr Akanksha Kotibhaskar.
- Ayurvedic and application inputs by Dr Ipsita Chatterjee.
- Nutrition and application inputs by Lovneet Batra.

Ginger and Garlic

- Ayurvedic inputs by Dr Akanksha Kotibhaskar.
- Nutrition and application inputs by Lovneet Batra.

Aloe Vera

- Super-shine aloe hair mask recipe by Dr Akanksha Kotibhaskar.
- Aloe skin-clearing lep recipe by Swati Kapoor, co-founder, SoulTree.
- Ayurvedic and application inputs by Dr Ipsita Chatterjee.
- Nutrition inputs by Lovneet Batra.

Turnips and Radishes

- Skin detox elixir recipe and application tips by Chef Sandeep Biswas.
- Nutrition inputs by Lovneet Batra.

Indian Gourds

- Glow-boosting elixir recipe and application inputs by Chef Sandeep Biswas.

- Sweet and tangy stuffed karela recipe by Anita Mathur, astrologer and homemaker, Delhi.
- Nutrition and application inputs by Lovneet Batra.
- Application inputs by Suparna Trikha.

Giloi

- Ayurvedic and application inputs by Dr Naresh Perumbuduri.
- Nutrition inputs by Lovneet Batra.

Wheatgrass

- Application inputs by Chef Sandeep Biswas.
- Nutrition and application inputs by Lovneet Batra.

Moong

- Exfoliating moong cleansing powder recipe by Dr Akanksha Kotibhaskar.
- Ayurvedic and application inputs by Dr Ipsita Chatterjee.
- Nutrition and application inputs by Lovneet Batra.
- Application inputs by Suparna Trikha.

PART III: RADIANCE

Moringa

- Ayurvedic and application inputs by Dr Naresh Perumbuduri.
- Nutrition inputs by Lovneet Batra.

Indian Berries

- Clarifying neem karela powder recipe and nutrition inputs by Lovneet Batra.

- Cooling falsa infusion recipe and Ayurvedic and application inputs by Dr Akanksha Kotibhaskar.
- Application inputs by Chef Sandeep Biswas.

Rose (Desi Gulab)

- Home-made rosewater recipe by Bubbles Singh, founder, Just B Au Naturel.
- Ayurvedic and application inputs by Dr Ipsita Chatterjee.
- Nutrition inputs by Lovneet Batra.
- Application inputs by Suparna Trikha.

Indian Greens

- Mom's mustard saag and Mom's bathua raita recipes by Veena Singh.
- Medicinal summer saag recipe by Kangan Badhwar, Kashmiri food expert, New Delhi.
- Ayurvedic and application inputs by Dr Jyotsna Makker.
- Nutrition and application inputs by Lovneet Batra.

Indian Seeds

- Ajwain period pain reliever recipe and nutrition and application inputs by Lovneet Batra.
- Methi bhringraj hair oil recipe by Swati Kapoor.
- Ayurvedic and application inputs by Dr Jyotsna Makker.

Marigold (Genda)

- Glow-boosting anti-acne mask recipe by Suparna Trikha.
- Ayurvedic inputs by Dr Ipsita Chatterjee.
- Nutrition and application inputs by Lovneet Batra.

Bitter Apricots

- Kashmiri skin balm and home-made apricot body wash recipes by Zahara Nedou, founder, Zahara Skincare.
- Nutrition and application inputs by Lovneet Batra.

PART IV: PEACE

Saffron (Kesar)

- Kashmiri saffron scrub recipe by Zahara Nedou.
- Ayurvedic inputs and application recipes by Dr Ipsita Chatterjee.
- Nutrition inputs by Lovneet Batra.

Holy Basil (Tulsi)

- Ayurvedic and application inputs by Dr Ipsita Chatterjee.
- Nutrition and application inputs by Lovneet Batra.

Gotu Kola

- Burmi saag recipe, Ayurvedic and application inputs by Dr Ipsita Chatterjee.
- Nutrition inputs by Lovneet Batra.

White Pumpkin (Petha)

- White pumpkin poriyal recipe by Chef Sandeep Biswas.
- White pumpkin South Indian kadhi recipe by Hema Gupta.
- Ayurvedic and application inputs by Dr Ipsita Chatterjee.
- Nutrition and application inputs by Lovneet Batra.

Bhringraj

- Bhringraj hair mask recipe by Suparna Trikha.
- Ayurvedic and application inputs by Dr Ipsita Chatterjee.
- Nutrition inputs by Lovneet Batra.

Jatamansi

- Calming bedtime drink recipe and Ayurvedic and application inputs by Dr Naresh Perumbuduri.
- Nutrition inputs by Lovneet Batra.

Camphor (Kapur)

- Ayurvedic and application inputs by Dr Ipsita Chatterjee.
- Nutrition inputs by Lovneet Batra.
- Application inputs by Suparna Trikha.

Sandalwood (Chandan)

- Ayurvedic and application inputs by Dr Ipsita Chatterjee.

A NOTE ON THE EXPERTS

Lovneet Batra

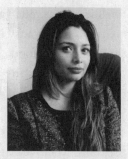

Lovneet is a Delhi-based nutritionist who believes that food is the most powerful form of medicine. She has counselled the Indian boxing, gymnastics, cycling and archery teams during the Commonwealth and Asian Games and is associated with Fortis Healthcare. She is also the founder of Nutrition by Lovneet and a visiting faculty at the Institute of Hotel Management (IHM), Pusa.

Dr Ipsita Chatterjee

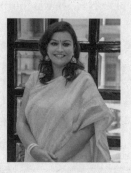

With a master's degree in Ayurvedic Rasashastra and Bhaishajya Kalpana (a branch dealing with Ayurveda pharmaceuticals and cosmetics), Ipsita is an Ayurvedic scientist who believes that true beauty is the light emanating from your own soul. She has been associated with the branded luxury Ayurveda beauty retail industry for over a decade and has an impressive track record in treating thousands of patients by providing wellness, diet and lifestyle consultations.

Sandeep Biswas

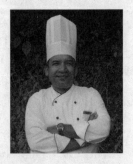

Chef Sandeep is one of the leading authorities on healthy cooking and has honed his skills by working in several wellness spas and also a Michelin-starred restaurant in London. He believes that food is thy medicine and medicine is thy food. As the former director, culinary, Ananda in the Himalayas, he brings a holistic balance to the book through a deep understanding of Ayurvedic cuisine and nutrition and culinary expertise. He has also worked at Four Seasons, Maldives, and Atmantan, Pune.

Dr Naresh Perumbuduri

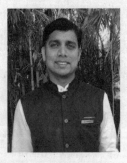

Dr Naresh was born in an Ayurveda family near Hyderabad where the traditional system was practised by four generations before him. After graduating from S.D.M. College of Ayurveda, Karnataka, he attained an MD in Ayurveda from Dr N.R.S. Ayurvedic Medical College, Andhra Pradesh. He has done extensive research in several psychological and physiological health issues. His specialization is in providing Ayurvedic solutions for autoimmune disorders. He is now a senior Ayurvedic physician at Ananda in the Himalayas.

Suparna Trikha

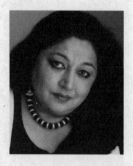

Suparna started India's first 100 per cent natural skin and hair centre that deals with beauty problems the natural way without using any chemicals or synthetics. She has been a regular beauty columnist with *The Telegraph*, *Savvy*, *Sahara*, *Sun* and *Grehlaxmi* and has given expert advice to leading magazines and newspapers like *Femina*, *Times of India*, *Hindustan Times*, *Cosmopolitan*, *Prevention* and *Marie Claire*, to name a few.

A NOTE ON THE AUTHOR

Vasudha Rai has worked as the beauty director for *Harper's Bazaar*, *Cosmopolitan* and *Women's Health*. Currently, she is a beauty columnist with *The Hindu* and regularly contributes to publications such as *Harper's Bazaar, Vogue, Elle* and *HT Mint*. Vasudha is a certified yoga teacher and teaches at The Yoga Studio, New Delhi. In her free time she writes on wellness, make-up and skincare on her blog *Vbeauty.co*.

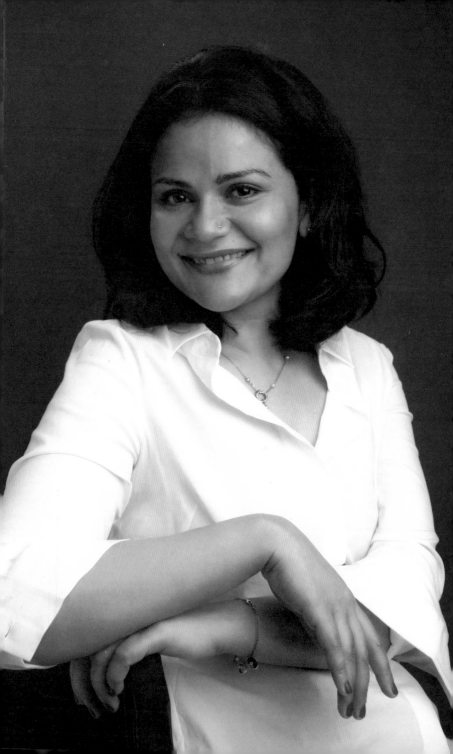

'A succinct guide to natural ingredients' *Mint Lounge*
'Why looking good is directly related to what you eat' *Harper's Bazaar*
'Atlas of natural beauty' *The Hindu Weekend*
'There's no questioning whether it really works' *Vogue*

Sixty Indian ingredients.
More than a 100 ways to use them.
Dive into the world of natural beauty.

Did you know that saffron can make you calmer? Or that tulsi protects you against pollution? Or that turnips and radishes help clear your complexion?

Whoever said that great skin is genetic has obviously never harnessed the power of beauty foods. While it is possible to fake great skin with make-up, you can be truly radiant only when you nourish your body from within. From basic garden-variety fruits and vegetables to potent Ayurvedic herbs, this book tells you what to eat to ensure that you stay beautiful inside and out.

Build strength and immunity, brighten and clarify your skin and achieve peace of mind with these powerful Indian remedies. These food combinations, recipes, face masks, oils and morning infusions will transform not just your skin but also your body and mind. After all, outer beauty is only a reflection of inner health.

Cover design by Meena Rajasekaran

FSC

Health

ISBN 978-0-143-44159-5

9 780143 441595
₹299
www.penguin.co.in

E-book available